W9-CEV-915

# THE BODY RESET DIET COOKBOOK

## ALSO BY HARLEY PASTERNAK

*The 5-Factor Diet*

*5-Factor Fitness*

*The 5-Factor World Diet*

*The Body Reset Diet*

# The
# BODY RESET
## Diet Cookbook

150 Recipes to Power Your Metabolism,
Blast Fat, and Shed Pounds in Just 15 Days

## HARLEY PASTERNAK, MSc

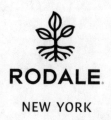

RODALE

NEW YORK

Copyright © 2014 by Bodiworx Health & Fitness, Inc.

All rights reserved.
Published in the United States by Rodale Books, an imprint of Random House, a
division of Penguin Random House LLC, New York.
rodalebooks.com

RODALE and the Plant colophon are registered trademarks of
Penguin Random House LLC.

Originally published in Canada by Penguin, an imprint of Penguin Canada Books
Inc., a division of Penguin Random House, in 2014.

Library of Congress Cataloging-in-Publication Data
Pasternak, Harley, author.
The body reset diet cookbook: 150 recipes to power your metabolism, blast fat,
and shed pounds in just 15 days / Harley Pasternak, MSc.
Includes index.
1. Reducing diets. 2. Reducing diets—recipes. 3. Cookbooks. I. Title.
RM222.2.P37752 2014          613.2'5
C2014-9004567

ISBN 978-0-593-23253-8
Ebook ISBN 978-1-62336-577-6

Printed in the United States of America

Photographs by Maya Visnyei Photography
Food stylist: Heather Shaw
Prop stylist: Catherine Doherty

10 9 8 7 6 5 4 3 2

First U.S. Edition

For my daughter, Liv

# Contents

# Introduction

Within a month of the release of *The Body Reset Diet* in 2013, I started to wake up every morning to an inbox full of messages from people I had never met before—people who were writing to me with the most incredible weight-loss stories you could imagine. These newly "lighter" individuals had successfully completed the first fifteen days of the Body Reset Diet and had dropped 10, 15, even 20 pounds in that time! They were exhilarated—they felt renewed, refreshed, reduced. They had actually *reset* their bodies, their palates, their digestion, and even their appetites.

Then the Twitter madness followed. From busy moms in Manitoba and Montana to household names like Kim (Kardashian), Jessica (Simpson), Megan (Fox), Hilary (Duff), and Robert (Pattinson), thousands of #bodyresetdiet messages were popping up everywhere.

I already knew that the Body Reset Diet—a structured and focused fifteen-day rapid eating plan that includes several delicious smoothies—was incredibly effective. I'd experienced the dramatic results myself, and I had seen many of my clients change their bodies in only days.

Although my previous books had been well received in more than thirty countries, I knew by the response to *The Body Reset Diet* that this book was unlike my others. *The Body Reset Diet* seemed to strike a deeper chord than other popular diet books, to a degree that surprised even me. Without any fancy marketing or promotional campaign, *The Body Reset Diet* caught fire, and it was all thanks to readers like you. You transformed your body with that book, then told your friends and co-workers about it, and they in turn told their families and neighbors about it, and soon my inbox was flooded with success stories. I am humbled and amazed by how effectively you spread the word about *The Body Reset Diet*, and I want to take this opportunity to thank all of you from the bottom of my heart.

As so many of you already know, the Body Reset Diet works because it's simple and it makes sense. You're never hungry. You always have time. And most important, the results come fast—and they stick.

For the last twenty-two years, I've always spoken about moderation, sustainability, and balance, and I've made sure everything I espouse is founded in hard science. Moreover, I understand how busy people are. I know that, regardless of how many studies back up a certain weight-loss method, if it isn't easy to follow, and doesn't deliver immediate results, it's not very useful.

I realized that most popular diets out there suffer from the same basic obstacles that get in the way of dieters' goals over and over again. I call these hurdles the Three Ts.

1. **Time:** Diets take too much time. You spend half your day weighing and measuring, then slicing and shredding, obscure

ingredients you've driven halfway across town to procure, and pretty soon you lose patience. The recipes in this book cover every major food group your body needs to thrive—and you can throw the meals together in mere minutes.

2. **Taste:** After several days of eating only baby food, or only cabbage soup, or only red meat, you (justifiably) want to go straight to the milkshake counter. Not so with *The Body Reset Diet Cookbook* recipes, which are as diverse as they are delicious. With tropical smoothies and spicy Asian wraps and everything in between, the recipes you'll find here offer tremendous variety, and countless options to keep your palate—and your stomach—satisfied.

3. **Transformation:** You have worked your butt off for two weeks straight, and you still can't zip up your jeans. Not fun. I can't blame you for wanting to quit. When you diet, you want results—and you want them now! Without measurable success, it's difficult to stay motivated. What makes the Body Reset Diet so successful is that you experience significant results in the first five days—and these results propel you to continue to achieve even more of your weight-loss goal.

The incredibly simple plan outlined in *The Body Reset Diet* delivers on all three fronts: it requires minimal preparation time, there is a wide variety of meals that all taste great, and you can expect to see results very quickly.

But the Body Reset Diet does more than give people the total body transformation that they aspire to achieve: it provides a healthy-eating springboard for years to come. If you combine the smoothies with what I call S-meals (S stands for *solid*, *simple*, and *single dish*, and includes salads, sandwiches, soups, stir-fries, and scrambles), you will feel amazing and you will love your body. And perhaps most important of all: you will never feel even the least bit deprived. You will begin making these meals because you want to lose weight, but you will continue making these meals because they're delicious and satisfying. It's all about the recipes.

I've written *The Body Reset Diet Cookbook* in response to the tremendous demand for more of the amazing smoothies and S-meals that made the original book such a hit. But you don't have to be a Body Reset veteran to get a ton of benefits from this book. I've also written this book for:

- those of you who haven't done the Body Reset Diet before but are curious what the buzz is all about,
- those of you who are looking for healthy recipes to supplement your everyday diet, and
- those of you who are already on the plan who have been asking me for more smoothies, more scrambles, more everything— here they are! I've been developing and perfecting these recipes for the past two years. You'll find 150 recipes here, half of them the smoothies that are the basis of the Body Reset Diet, and half of them the delicious S-meals that are so quick and convenient to prepare.

Although the smoothies are made with a wide range of ingredients, all of them, and the S-meals, adhere to the same basic nutritional profile. They're all approximately 300 calories, and they all have about

20 grams of protein and 10 grams of fiber. Every time you prepare one of these meals, you can rest assured that what you're about to eat is balanced and nutritious and will keep you feeling satiated for several hours. Unlike a juice cleanse or some extreme fast, you are not cheating your body of any essential nutrients when you follow the Body Reset Diet.

And although every single one of these recipes is nutritionally interchangeable, the sheer quantity of them means that you will never get bored, which is key to the success of any diet. If you combine these 150 recipes with the ones already available in *The Body Reset Diet* and my previous three books, *5-Factor Fitness*, *The 5-Factor Diet*, and *The 5-Factor World Diet*, you will have an even bigger selection of healthy meals to choose from. The recipes in this cookbook will help you lose weight and make eating right hassle-free and even fun.

"Wow. I never thought I could feel this good!
I actually crave the Body Reset Diet smoothies
when I get hungry. Your whole approach is
a wonderful, refreshing change from the
pushy, unattainable demands of most
health professionals. Thank you. I am down
13 pounds of the 35 I would like to lose,
but to be honest, it's not the weight that
now motivates me, it's the amazing
way my WHOLE body feels.
I feel alive—no more sluggishness!"

Teri
Nepean, Ontario

"I live for Harley's smoothies! They are so easy to make, help me feel full, and taste incredible!"

—Kim Kardashian

# PART 1

## Understanding the Body Reset Diet

# CHAPTER ONE

# The Body Reset Diet Explained

Whether you're starting from Day 1 on the fifteen-day Body Reset or just enhancing your everyday diet with these recipes, I want to go over the fundamentals of how this diet works so that you can get the most out of the recipes in this book regardless of your goals.

Firstly, as with my 5-Factor diet, I recommend eating five times a day to rev up your metabolism. Eating frequent small meals is far better for the body than the feast-and-famine cycles so many dieters endure. In the Body Reset, you'll be eating three meals a day (some combination of smoothies and S-meals) along with two simple snacks, which I call C-snacks, for reasons I'll explain shortly.

It's important to bear in mind that not all calories are created equal. While every meal in this book has roughly the same calorie count (about 300), what you're eating matters just as much as its

## Grazing versus Gorging

Researchers at the University of Toronto found that men who ate three large meals a day had higher insulin levels than those who "nibbled," or grazed, on seventeen small meals. This study and similar ones demonstrated that "grazing" on smaller amounts of food more frequently does a better job of priming our bodies to burn fat more effectively than "gorging" on larger quantities of food two or three times a day.

calorie content: a 300-calorie scoop of ice cream, for example, is just not nutritionally equivalent to a filling 300-calorie egg white, veggie, and ham scramble with a side of whole wheat toast. The first gives you a sugar high that leaves you tired and hungry half an hour later; the second fills you up and fuels you for hours afterward. Make every calorie work for you.

One way to do this is to ensure that everything you eat—every single meal and snack—contains both

- fiber, and
- protein.

I'll explain later why getting these two elements in at every meal is crucial for controlling your appetite (and, not so coincidentally, your weight).

"Having smoothies twice a day,
two snacks, and a meal at dinner has
become a lifestyle for me. Finally, after trying just
about every diet there is (which all state that "it needs
to be a lifestyle change"), the Body Reset Diet is a
lifestyle change for me. Thank you, Harley, for
your help in making me a healthier person."

Darlene P. (Calgary, Alberta)

## The Body Reset Diet in Three Easy Phases

The Body Reset Diet consists of three distinct five-day phases lasting a total of fifteen days. You'll be eating five—yes, five!—times a day, alternating nutritious, delicious, and filling smoothies with snacks and S-meals, all of which you will be able to prepare yourself in remarkably little time.

Throughout the Body Reset Diet (and for the rest of your life), you'll be moving constantly, logging a total of at least 10,000 steps, or about five miles (8 km), every single day. *The Body Reset Diet* also contains detailed instructions on some quick, simple strength-training exercises for you to incorporate into your daily routine. But first and foremost, we need to change the sedentary lifestyle that is responsible for so many of our health problems these days.

## TIP

Think of these recipes as a template. Feel free to improvise with your own favorite ingredients and flavors, as long as you're sticking to the basic nutritional profile. I encourage you to tweak some of the smoothie recipes to suit your tastes, subbing in kale for spinach, or pears for apples—whatever works for you.

## Is Sitting the New Smoking?

An Australian study published in 2012 compared sitting to smoking, with some truly scary results. The study found that for every hour of TV people watch (presumably while seated), their life span is shortened by 22 minutes. Every cigarette people smoke, by contrast, shortens their life by about 11 minutes.

Get moving! Even if, like so many of us, you have a desk job, you should make a concerted effort to simply get up and move whenever you can. You'll be shocked by how good you look and feel.

# The Breakdown

If you're new to the Body Reset Diet and embarking on the fifteen-day kick start to this plan, here's how it works.

## Phase I

In Phase I, between Days 1 and 5, you'll be drinking three smoothies a day and eating two snacks. This sounds intense, but remember that these fiber-packed smoothies are as filling as they are delicious. From the very first day of the plan, you need to start walking 10,000 steps a day, using a pedometer to track your steps.

### PHASE I DIET
3 smoothies
2 C-snacks

### PHASE I EXERCISE
Walk 10,000 steps a day

## Phase II

In Phase II, Days 6 through 10, you will continue to eat five times a day, but instead of three smoothies you'll have two smoothies and one S-meal, plus two C-snacks.

### PHASE II DIET
2 smoothies
1 S-meal (at the meal of your choosing)
2 C-snacks

# C-Snacks

Twice a day, every day for fifteen days, you'll eat **C-snacks**, so called because they tend to be crunchy, such as cut veggies (like celery, carrots, or broccoli) or crackers with a high fiber content (which I define as at least 5 grams of fiber per 100 calories). Like everything you eat, the fiber in C-snacks must always be paired with a protein. A good C-snack might be

- Crunchy cut veggies with nut butter
- Crackers with hummus

Most C-snacks take no time to make. See page 28 for a list of suggested snacks, which should all be approximately 150 calories.

## PHASE II EXERCISE

Walk 10,000 steps a day
Five-minute strength-training circuit, three days a week

For more detail on the types of strength-training exercises you need to be doing, please refer to *The Body Reset Diet*, which contains illustrated step-by-step descriptions of the exercises that you can do in any room in your house, with little or no equipment.

## Phase III

You're almost there! Phase III covers the last five days of the kick-start plan, when you'll go down to one smoothie a day, plus two S-meals and your usual two C-snacks.

## PHASE III DIET

1 smoothie

2 S-meals (at the meals of your choosing)

2 C-snacks

## PHASE III EXERCISE

Walk 10,000 steps a day

Five-minute strength-training circuit, five days a week

## The Rest of Your Life

Once you've completed the fifteen-day Body Reset, you should continue walking 10,000 steps a day—yep, every day for the rest of your life. You should also continue alternating two five-minute exercise circuits five days a week. You can gradually increase this to three circuits at every session.

## The Free Meal

At your twice-weekly free meal (only for the "Rest of Your Life" phase), you can eat or drink whatever you want. Do you have a special date night planned, or a Saturday lunch with old friends? Then indulge to your heart's content. Or stick to the basic outlines of your usual diet, but enjoy a dessert, or a few drinks with your meal—it's up to you. These two weekly meals are "free" because they consist of whatever you want them to.

As for your diet, just keep going! One smoothie, two S-meals, and two C-snacks every day, with one big difference: now you get two "free meals" a week where you break all the rules … as long as you return to your good habits by the next meal.

You can stick with this "maintenance phase" of the plan for weeks or even years. The two free meals mean you never feel deprived—and the delicious smoothies and S-meals mean you're always satisfied.

"I got back to the gym in December, hit it really hard, and tried a bunch of different diets: Weight Watchers, calorie counting, and many others. Nothing worked, and I was tired and frustrated. I picked up *The Body Reset Diet* and I felt like the light came on. Everything you said about the crazy gym classes, working out so hard and then sitting on the couch all afternoon, the food obsessions about what to eat and not to eat—it all just made sense to me. I have so much more time not being at the gym for two hours a day, and my family is so happy! I feel so positive about this change. Thank you for helping me!"

Susan O. (Hinesburg, Vermont)

# The Benefits of Blending

Regardless of whether you're planning to make the recipes in this book consistently or just occasionally, you will need a blender. You can't make smoothies without one.

Blending is a fantastic way to prepare food, for many reasons. First off, it's easy. You don't need an oven or a timer or any culinary expertise. No matter how crunched for time you are, you can throw some ingredients in a blender and switch it on. Voila, in ninety seconds max, you have a delicious and balanced meal.

If you invest in a high-end blender like the Vitamix or Blendtec (which I recommend if you plan on making these smoothies regularly), prep work is even more minimal. You can throw whole apples or almonds right into the blender and within seconds they'll be transformed into hearty, filling smoothies. Blending is also super convenient for those who are constantly on the go: you can make blended drinks in advance and take them to work with you—just refrigerate them and shake well before serving.

# The Body Reset Diet Every Day

You can always return to Phase I of the diet if you want to lose weight fast. Or, if you wish to maintain your weight, you could drink a smoothie every morning, or take your favorite S-meal sandwich to work once a week. Whether you use these recipes for every meal or just every once in a while, this cookbook will play a big role in helping

## The Fiber Connection

Perhaps most important of all for our purposes, a blender makes it easy to get more healthy ingredients into your diet. Once you start drinking these smoothies, you'll find that you're consuming far more fruits and vegetables than ever before (often without even noticing they're there). And unlike sugar-filled juices, blended drinks contain a ton of fiber, which is essential for

• losing weight
• maintaining bowel health
• satisfying your appetite

I cannot emphasize enough the importance of a fiber-rich diet when it comes to healthy living, which is why I recommend that everyone consume at least 40 grams of fiber a day. You need fiber in every meal, and the Body Reset smoothies are packed with it.

you look and feel your best for the rest of your life. Your energy levels will increase, your mood will improve, and you will watch in awe as the pounds melt right off.

"Originally, I was going to do the Body Reset Diet
by myself, but as I was reading the first few chapters
of the book, I knew this was something that could work
for both me and my husband. Jason was skeptical at first,
but the more I told him about it, the more he was on board.
He started the plan at 499.8 pounds and has lost 14.
I started at 276 and have lost 7 pounds.

"We have obviously tried other plans and they just
didn't work for us. We have both been having some health
problems—high blood pressure, for example—and knew we had
to make a change. Both of us are 32 and are too young to be
having health issues like this. Finding *The Body Reset Diet* when
we did was perfect timing. We were ready for a change, a major
one, but it had to be healthy and something that would teach
us how to eat and how to maintain a healthy lifestyle.

"Staying on plan has helped our wallet, too! No restaurant
food for fifteen days is saving us money and showing us
how easy it can be to eat at home. While my husband
is excellent in the kitchen, I am not, so having
easy-to-prepare meals really helps me out!"

Nahtanha K. (Erie, Pennsylvania)

# CHAPTER TWO

# Stocking Your Body Reset Kitchen

All right, now let's go shopping! It's time to dump the junk and to fill your kitchen with healthy, good-for-you ingredients. I always recommend stocking up on dried goods (such as beans and grains) and frozen foods (especially fruits and vegetables) so that you will always have healthy food on hand, even on the days when you're too busy, or just too tired, to hit the store. You do NOT want to get in a situation where the only food in your house is your child's old Halloween candy. If you keep unhealthy items in the house, it's much harder to resist them.

Keep nutritious ingredients around and you'll be more likely to toss a healthy meal together, especially when you're pressed for time.

The following section is broken down into the essential ingredients for smoothies, S-meals, and C-snacks. It is pretty comprehensive, and you don't need to buy everything at once. Your own personal shopping list will depend on whether you're doing the full-on fifteen-day plan or just supplementing your diet with a few healthier meals a week. What follows is a "greatest hits" selection of the ingredients that appear most often in the recipes in this cookbook.

"My husband and I moved out to the burbs to be close to my new job. We bought a car and no longer walk everywhere, and we gained quite a bit of weight in just a few months. Despite trying to eat healthy, we were not able to shed the pounds.

"We just finished our fifteen-day program and we've both lost over 9 pounds each! More than that is the fact that I feel ten years younger: I sleep better, wake up refreshed, and have more energy during the day. Your recipes are fantastic! (Our favorite is the Coconut Curry Chicken.) This started as a diet, but it has become a lifestyle. It has simplified the processes of grocery shopping and food preparation, and has significantly reduced the grocery bill."

Jim and Mick Z. (North York, Ontario)

# Smoothie Essentials

All the smoothies in this book consist of four basic categories of ingredients.

**Category 1: LIQUID BASE** is the core of every Body Reset smoothie: you may notice the blender doesn't work quite as well without it. Depending on the calorie count and nutritional profile of the recipe, you can use either water or one of the following bases.

## LIQUID BASE SUGGESTIONS

**Organic dairy milk:** I am a huge fan of dairy milk. High in protein, calcium, vitamin D, phosphorus, and other essential nutrients, what's not to love? Its high calcium content can also expedite weight loss. I prefer skim, or fat-free, milk, but 1% is also OK.

**Nondairy milk:** Some people have trouble digesting the natural sugar in dairy milk (lactose), some are allergic to the protein in milk (casein), and still others choose to avoid animal products. There are plenty of acceptable alternatives to dairy milk (provided they're low in fat and sugar), including soy, rice, almond, hemp, and oat milks.

## TIP

When shopping for nondairy milks, always read the nutritional profiles and avoid any milks with more than 2 grams of fat and/or 10 grams of sugars per serving.

Category 2: PROTEIN consists of the building blocks of life and as such is essential to every meal. Protein is particularly important for building muscle, and the more muscle we have, the more calories we burn all day, even at rest. That's why maintaining lean muscle mass is so critical to sustaining weight loss. Also, because the body burns more energy digesting protein than any other food, protein is a fat-burning double whammy. In fact, studies show that people who eat protein at every meal consistently lose more weight than those who don't. Because we can't store protein—we must either use it or excrete it—we need to consume a consistent supply throughout the day.

## PROTEIN SUGGESTIONS

**Nonfat plain Greek yogurt:** Yogurt is a great source of calcium and vitamin D as well as two kinds of protein: casein and whey. I prefer Greek yogurt to regular yogurt because it's higher in protein and lower in sugar and lactose, with roughly the same calorie count. And studies show that high-calcium foods like Greek yogurt directly aid in weight-loss efforts.

**Protein powder:** I love the convenience of protein powder because it doesn't need refrigeration. Protein powders come in many varieties, but not all are created equal—some are missing amino acids, some are more difficult to digest, and some might contain allergenic ingredients.

## TIP

Whey protein is my preferred type of protein powder. Read the label and make sure that what you buy has less than 2 grams of fat and 2 grams of sugar and derives at least 90 percent of its calories from protein.

Other good options:

- Whey concentrate
- Egg white (albumin)
- Whey-casein blend
- Pea protein
- Brown rice protein
- Soy protein

**Tofu:** Tofu is another great source of protein that goes well in smoothies. I prefer the silken and soft varieties. Make sure to purchase low-fat varieties.

## Category 3: HIGH-FIBER FRUITS AND VEGETABLES are

central to a healthy diet. Both are carbohydrates, but there's a big difference between bad carbohydrates (white breads, pastas, and simple sugars) and the good ones like fruits and vegetables. The recipes in *The Body Reset Diet Cookbook* focus on complex carbohydrates, which take the body a long time to digest and don't cause spikes in blood sugar levels. Body Reset–approved carbs also tend to be high in fiber. Fiber helps move food through the body and facilitates weight loss. Carbohydrates in this expansive category include pretty much all fruits and vegetables.

## FRUIT AND VEGETABLE SUGGESTIONS

All berries

Apples

Pears

Vegetables

Almost all vegetables are good, especially spinach and other leafy greens. Leafy greens are high in fiber and extremely calorie-efficient—meaning you get a lot of bang for your nutritional buck, which is key when dieting—and they're packed with all sorts of antioxidants and anti-inflammatory agents.

Category 4: HEALTHY FATS are a fundamental part of every Body Reset meal. Your body needs fat, protein, and carbohydrates—without these macronutrients, you can't function properly. Fat supplies you with energy and helps your body absorb essential vitamins. Fat is also crucial for your hormones, nerves, reproductive system, skin, and last but not least, your brain. Your brain especially needs the healthy fats found in omega-3 and omega-6 fatty acids, which our bodies do not produce—we can get them only through food. Most of us get too many omega-6s and not enough omega-3s, which is why the Body Reset Diet recipes contain higher concentrations of omega-3s.

# Good Fats versus Bad Fats

Many of us are frightened of the word *fat*, but there's a big difference between the "good," or healthy, fats we eat in the Body Reset Diet and the "bad" fats associated with heart disease and other illnesses. Bad fats include the saturated fats found in many animal products, such as red meat, poultry skin, whole milk, butter, and egg yolks. The worst fats of all are the trans fats, or hydrogenated fats, found mostly in commercially processed foods like doughnuts, cookies, and fried foods. While it's fine to eat small amounts of saturated fats, you should never eat these artificial trans fats.

## HEALTHY FAT SUGGESTIONS

**Nuts:** You can add any kind of nut you'd like to your smoothies. Cashews, macadamia nuts, pecans, and walnuts are all good in small quantities. Almonds, which have been shown to expedite weight loss, are a particular favorite of mine.

**Seeds:** Flaxseeds are a wonderful source of omega-3 fatty acids (as well as fiber), and they have a wonderful nutty flavor that tastes great in most smoothies. For some variety, try chia seeds, sunflower seeds, or pumpkin seeds.

> ## TIP
>
> If you're making smoothies ahead of time, don't add the seeds until right before you're ready to drink. Seeds expand when they're exposed to liquid. If you don't drink the smoothie right away, it will become too thick to drink.

**Avocado:** Avocados keep your skin supple and beautiful and can help your body absorb essential nutrients. Like nuts and various vegetable oils, particularly olive oil, avocado is a great source of monounsaturated fat, a "good" fat that can decrease your overall cholesterol level and lower your risk of heart disease.

You can also toss into your smoothies what I call accent ingredients. One of these is cinnamon, which, in addition to giving a flavor boost to any smoothie, can help regulate blood sugar and speed up metabolism.

## Smoothie Shopping List

If you're planning to do the fifteen-day Body Reset Diet, you'll need to load up on a variety of smoothie ingredients. Luckily, many of the necessary staples aren't perishable; you can keep them in your freezer or pantry until you're ready to put them in the blender. Also, you do not need all of the following ingredients, even for the full fifteen-day Body Reset. I'm just giving you all your options in each of the four ingredient categories.

# #1 LIQUID BASES

Organic skim dairy milk

OR …

Almond milk

Soy milk

Oat milk

Rice milk

Hemp milk

# #2 PROTEIN

Protein powder (whey, albumin, casein, whey-casein blend, soy, pea, rice, hemp)

Nonfat plain Greek yogurt

Tofu (low-fat)

# #3 HIGH-FIBER FRUITS AND VEGETABLES

## Fresh

Apples

Limes

Oranges

Spinach

Bananas and grapes, commonly used in the recipes, are not considered high-fiber fruits. They are added more for sweetness.

## Frozen

| | |
|---|---|
| Blackberries | Raspberries |
| Blueberries | Strawberries |

## #4 HEALTHY FATS

Almonds or almond butter

Avocados

Chia seeds (whole or ground)

Flaxseeds (whole or ground)

Peanuts or peanut butter

## #5 ACCENT INGREDIENTS

Cinnamon (apple, pear, banana)

Ginger (pear, apple, cucumber, carrot)

Mint (melon, citrus, berries)

Lemon (apple, greens, carrot)

Lime (mango, pineapple, berries)

Vanilla (peach, almond, coconut)

# S-Meal Essentials

The "S" in S-meals stands for *solid* (the opposite of smoothies), and also for *simple* and *single dish*. Types of S-meals are

- salads
- soups
- stir-fries
- scrambles
- sandwiches

Since S-meals adhere to the same basic nutritional profile as the smoothies in this book, they also contain similar categories of ingredients. Every S-meal will have

- protein
- high-fiber fruits, vegetables, and grains
- healthy fats
- accent ingredients

## Category 1: PROTEIN

Unlike the case with carbohydrates and fats, your body is not very good at storing protein, so you have to get small hits of it throughout the day. Studies show that people who eat small amounts of protein with each meal are leaner than those who don't.

**Eggs and egg whites:** While a whole egg has long been the gold standard as "the perfect protein," yolks have a high caloric load and also a lot of saturated fat. Egg whites are a great option for those wanting lots of high-quality protein without too many calories.

**Seafood:** From salmon to scallops and tilapia to shrimp, seafood is loaded with high-quality protein and healthy fats. Try to minimize your intake of high-mercury fish such as tuna and swordfish. Focus on smaller fish, freshwater fish, and shellfish.

**Red meat:** Packed with protein and tons of iron, red meat can be part of a healthy diet as long as it's relatively lean and not overcooked. (Overcooking lean meat will make it very dry and therefore less appetizing.) Beef is the most common red meat, but alternative proteins like bison and ostrich are delicious, leaner options that are gaining in popularity.

**Tofu and tempeh:** These extremely easy-to-use vegetarian sources of protein are made from soybeans. Delicious "animal protein" substitutes, also made from soy protein, are available in a wide range of options, including veggie dogs, bacon, and burgers.

**Poultry:** Chicken and turkey are great protein options. Avoid eating the skin, which is high in saturated fat, and opt for the breast meat whenever possible.

## VEGETARIAN AND VEGAN PROTEIN OPTIONS

**Beans and legumes:** Beans and lentils, a favorite food of vegetarians, are cheap and incredibly versatile. I recommend canned beans and lentils because they are far easier to prepare. Beans and legumes are high in all three food categories (protein, fiber, and healthy fat), so don't let their placement in the protein section stop you from using them in the other groups as well.

*Lentils:* Canned lentils are a perfect addition to soups and salads, and they make delicious spreads when puréed.

*Black beans:* Stock up on canned black beans, which add a punch of flavor—and a whole lot of fiber—to many recipes.

*Chickpeas:* Chickpeas, or garbanzo beans, are extremely high in protein, zinc, and folate, and of course fiber.

*Pinto beans:* Pinto beans have it all: fiber, folate, magnesium, and potassium. They're delicious in chili.

*White beans:* Cannellini are a variety of white kidney bean used in Italian cooking. They have a delicate, mild flavor and are great in soups. Other types of white beans, such as navy, Great Northern, and black-eyed peas, offer similar nutritional benefits—mainly high fiber—and are a great alternative to meat protein.

## Category 2: HIGH-FIBER FRUITS, VEGETABLES, AND GRAINS

If proteins are the building blocks of the "me" machine, then fibrous carbohydrates like fruits, vegetables, and whole grains are the fuel.

**Fruits:** Choose fruits that have edible skin or seeds or citrus fruits. These kinds of fruits do not make your blood sugar surge and tend to be lower in calories.

| | |
|---|---|
| Apples | Nectarines |
| Berries (all) | Oranges |
| Cherries | Peaches |
| Grapefruits | Pears |
| Kiwifruits | Plums |

**Vegetables:** The rule with vegetables is … there is no rule. For the most part, eat as much as you want. The few exceptions are vegetables high in starch (such as potatoes) or sugar (such as beets and corn). Some good staple vegetables to keep around include

| | |
|---|---|
| Bell peppers | Onions |
| Cucumber | Romaine lettuce |
| Garlic | Spinach |
| Green peas | Sweet potatoes |
| Kale | Tomatoes |

**Grains:** The healthiest cultures in the world all include some kind of grain in their diets. Don't let the passé "carb-free" diet fad scare you away from these nutrient-dense, fibrous foods.

*Quinoa*: Quinoa looks and acts a lot like rice and other cereal grains, but it's actually a seed. It's high in protein, delicious, and incredibly easy to prepare.

*Wild rice*: Wild rice has a nutty taste and is high in fiber, protein, and lysine—and is low-fat to boot!

*Barley*: Barley is a great-tasting alternative to rice or pasta that's high in both fiber and protein. It's extremely versatile and filling.

*High-fiber bread*: Bread is not the enemy! Just avoid white bread. Choose high-fiber whole-grain bread with fewer than 100 calories and at least 4 grams of fiber per slice.

*High-fiber tortillas*: You can find high-fiber tortillas made from corn or whole wheat at almost every grocery store.

## Category 3: HEALTHY FATS

Fats are essential to your health. They serve to fuel your nervous system and create your hormones. Research has shown that eating certain healthy fats can actually help burn off unwanted visceral fat (the stuff around our organs).

Olive oil
Nuts (almonds, peanuts, cashews, etc.)
Nut oils
Nut butters (all-natural, with no added oils or sugars)
Seeds (sesame, chia, flax, pumpkin)
Avocados
Olives

## Category 4: ACCENT INGREDIENTS

**Herbs and spices:** Fresh herbs are a great source of antioxidants and add a boost of flavor to foods without extra calories. Keep their dried counterparts around in case you run out—they also have great benefits. The herbs and spices we use most often in this cookbook are

### Fresh
Basil
Chives
Cilantro
Parsley
Thyme

### Dried
Cinnamon
Oregano

**Condiments:** Condiments are another great way to add major flavor without a lot of extra calories. Try to stick to options that aren't too high in calories (balsamic vinegar, lemon juice, Worcestershire and hot sauces) and those containing healthy fats (such as olive oil).

# C-Snack Essentials

C-snacks ("C" stands for *crunchy*) are less structured than the smoothies and S-meals: you find what you like and you go with it. But there are certain basic guidelines. All C-snacks should contain no more than 150 calories and

- at least 5 grams of fiber
- at least 5 grams of protein
- less than 10 grams of sugar

Whenever you buy packaged foods, read the nutrition information to ensure that they contain fiber and/or protein and have fewer than 150 calories per serving. Here are some examples of great protein- and fiber-combining C-snacks:

- high-fiber crackers with turkey slices
- carrot and zucchini wedges with hummus
- skim milk latte and a few almonds
- apple slices
- air-popped popcorn
- Greek yogurt with berries
- The Good Bean bars
- edamame

Play around with variations—they're endless. You're limited only by your own creativity!

"I consider myself a pretty active person. I go
to the gym at least three times a week and eat a
pretty healthy diet. The problem is, I was struggling
with the last 10 to 15 pounds. No matter how much
cardio I did, I had definitely hit a plateau. Then I
saw your book. I started the diet the next morning
with the Apple Pie Smoothie. Wow! So simple and
yummy! By the next morning, I was running out of
bed, had so much energy, and actually felt better.
By the fifth day, I was bouncing off walls, I looked
leaner, and the belly fat I thought was a part of me
since my cesarean section was almost gone. I told
my husband that this diet has become my new way
of life. Ten pounds have come off so far and I am still
seeing changes. I want to thank you again for this
book—with its tasty and realistic recipes, I feel like
I have finally conquered the battle of the bulge."

Tanya L. (St. Albert, Alberta)

# Complete Pantry for the
# Body Reset Diet Recipes

Here are some suggestions and ideas for ingredients, health, and cooking associated with the recipes in this book.

**Oils:** cooking oil spray (vegetable and extra-virgin olive oil), extra-virgin olive oil, grapeseed, canola (or other vegetable oils), sesame oil (for Asian dishes), nut oils (for desserts, dressings), infused oils (for appetizers, salads, garnishing)

There are many oils to choose from when cooking. The type of cuisine and cooking method will help to determine which is best suited. Use spray oil in frying or roasting pans to keep things light. Sesame oil works wonderfully in Asian and some Mediterranean, African, and Middle Eastern dishes. Nut and infused oils are a nice added flavor for salad dressings. Many oils, such as extra-virgin olive, have been linked to a lower risk of heart disease and high blood pressure, among other health benefits.

**Vinegars:** white wine, red wine, sherry, balsamic, apple cider, rice wine, other fruit vinegars

Stock up on a variety of vinegars for different flavors and cuisines. Balsamic is great for marinating or making salad dressings, whereas rice wine vinegar can be used in Asian-inspired recipes. Apple cider vinegar can aid in settling an upset stomach and can even supply a boost of energy.

**Herbs and spices:** allspice, basil, cardamom, cayenne pepper, chili powder, chipotle chili (ground), chives, cilantro, cinnamon, cloves, coriander, cumin, curry powder, fennel seeds, ginger (dried and fresh), garlic powder, herbes de Provence, Italian seasoning, lemon pepper, marjoram, nutmeg, oregano, paprika (regular and smoked), parsley, black pepper, hot pepper flakes, rosemary, sage, salt (kosher, sea, flaky, smoked), sesame seeds, tarragon, thyme

Having a well-stocked spice rack means you aren't stuck using the same old seasonings dish after dish. Look for fresh herbs when available, or grow your own on your kitchen windowsill. Many herbs and spices contain high amounts of antioxidants, can lower blood sugar and cholesterol, and can even inhibit the growth of cancer cells.

**Baking supplies:** Ingredients like oats, flaxseeds, and bran contain soluble fiber, which helps to lower "bad" cholesterol levels.

**Bread:** high-fiber bread, low-carb high-fiber tortillas, whole-grain pitas, whole-grain baguette, reduced-calorie bread, bread crumbs (panko, whole-grain, Italian, gluten-free)

Bread products labeled high-fiber or whole-grain contain added fiber in the form of wheat bran, oat bran, soy, or seeds. In addition to fiber, whole-grain breads contain protein, vitamins, antioxidants, and minerals and have been linked to reducing the risk of heart disease.

**Pasta, noodles, grains:** shirataki type, whole-grain (quinoa, spelt, etc.), mung bean (high in fiber and protein)

Try out the many great alternatives to regular pasta. Choosing alternative noodles, such as shirataki, allows you to create recipes that are satisfying, delicious, and full of nutrition without added calories. Quinoa, barley, brown rice, and spelt are delicious grains that provide complex carbohydrates, amino acids, and protein.

**Dairy/nondairy goods:** Dairy products like milk, cheese, and yogurt are rich in vitamin D and calcium, which promote strong bones and reduce the risk of osteoporosis. Choosing low-fat or fat-free dairy items can help keep cholesterol levels healthy and control calorie intake.

Nondairy alternatives can also add protein and calcium to your diet. Many types of nondairy milks are available at the grocery store (coconut, almond, hemp, hazelnut, soy). Choose an unsweetened variety to ensure you're not adding any additional calories or sugar to your diet.

**Sweeteners:** agave syrup/nectar, blackstrap molasses (nutrients), coconut palm sugar (nutrients), honey

Using sweeteners that are low on the glycemic index, such as agave, will help moderate blood sugar levels and avoid the "sugar crash." Compared to traditional sugar, these alternatives have lower calorie counts and some even contain vitamins and minerals. Honey contains health boosters like flavonoids and antioxidants.

**Proteins:** tofu, tempeh (with flax, etc.), skinless chicken or turkey breast, lean beef, fish/shellfish, lean pork

Choosing meat and poultry cuts that are lean and low in fat will allow you to get adequate protein without adding undesired fat and calories. Fish provides a high amount of protein as well as omega-3 fatty acids, which reduce inflammation and keep your heart healthy. Tofu and tempeh are great vegetarian alternatives and have been shown to help lower "bad" cholesterol. Along with providing protein, soy products are a good source of vitamin E and calcium.

**Vegetables and legumes (high in fiber and protein):** Legumes are a great option for vegetarians. They are naturally low in fat and high in protein. They are a complex carbohydrate, providing plenty of fiber, and they are filling, which can help maintain a healthy weight. Vegetables that are high in protein and fiber are essential for weight management. Studies have shown that diets rich in high-fiber vegetables such as cauliflower and broccoli are linked to cancer prevention. Dark leafy greens not only provide calcium and iron but also can help provide relief from digestive issues.

**Fruits:** Fruits that are high in fiber act to slow the absorption of sugar, which is beneficial for those with diabetes. Bulking your diet with high-protein, high-fiber fruits can increase a sense of fullness while maintaining a lower caloric intake.

**Flavor boosters:** canned chipotle chilies in adobo sauce, Worcestershire sauce, Sriracha sauce, hot sauce (such as Tabasco), Old Bay seasoning, Cajun seasoning, taco seasoning, miso paste, fish sauce, soy sauce (low-sodium), mirin

These types of ingredients can help turn an ordinary dish into an extraordinary one. They often provide that extra touch of authenticity that brings out the flavors of a regional or specialty dish. Getting to know the special ingredients used in various cuisines can be exciting and educational, and can take your culinary repertoire to new heights.

"The Body Reset Diet makes healthy eating easier. The smoothies are simple to prepare, taste great, and are the perfect breakfast or snack when I'm on the go."

—Amanda Seyfried

# PART 2

## The Body Reset Diet Recipes

# SMOOTHIES

## White Smoothies

## Red Smoothies

## Green Smoothies

# Other Smoothies

# Apple Coconut Smoothie

It is important to use unsweetened coconut milk beverage. Most store-bought coconut milks are loaded with sugar and extra calories.  **SERVES 1**

¾ cup (175 mL) unsweetened coconut milk beverage

1 cup (250 mL) chopped peeled cored apple

1 small frozen banana, chopped

1 serving unsweetened protein powder

½ teaspoon (2 mL) grated fresh ginger

1½ teaspoons (7 mL) chia seeds

4 ice cubes

Place ingredients in a blender in the order listed. Blend until desired consistency is reached, adding water to thin out if necessary.

---

**MODIFIED VERSION**

For men or those 170 pounds (77 kg) and up, increase ingredients by one-third.

---

**Nutritional Information (per serving)**

Calories 330  •  Carbs 46 grams  •  Protein 25 grams  •  Fat 7 grams  •  Fiber 8 grams

# Hawaiian Smoothie

I created this smoothie when I was living in Hawaii. While there, I also learned that Spam—the canned "meat" product—is a regional favorite! **SERVES 1**

½ cup (125 mL) water (or more, depending on preferred texture)

½ cup (125 mL) unsweetened coconut milk beverage

½ cup (125 mL) frozen chopped mango

¼ cup (60 mL) frozen chopped pineapple

½ small frozen banana, chopped

½ cup (125 mL) chopped cored unpeeled apple

1 serving unsweetened protein powder

1 tablespoon (15 mL) chia seeds

Ice cubes (optional)

Place ingredients in a blender in the order listed. Add ice if preferred. Blend until desired consistency is reached, adding more water to thin out if necessary.

---

## MODIFIED VERSION
For men or those 170 pounds (77 kg) and up, increase ingredients by one-third.

---

### Nutritional Information (per serving)

Calories 360 • Carbs 50 grams • Protein 26 grams • Fat 8 grams • Fiber 9 grams

# Banana Spice Smoothie

I love this smoothie. Pumpkin spice, banana, and apple. Yes, please! **SERVES 1**

½ cup (125 mL) unsweetened almond milk

1 medium frozen banana, chopped

1 cup (250 mL) chopped cored unpeeled apple

½ teaspoon (2 mL) pumpkin pie spice

1 serving unsweetened protein powder

1 tablespoon (15 mL) chia seeds

Ice cubes (optional)

Place ingredients in a blender in the order listed. Add ice if preferred. Blend until desired consistency is reached, adding water to thin out if necessary.

---

**MODIFIED VERSION**

For men or those 170 pounds (77 kg) and up, increase ingredients by one-third.

---

**Nutritional Information (per serving)**

Calories 326  •  Carbs 44 grams  •  Protein 26 grams  •  Fat 7 grams  •  Fiber 9 grams

# A(pricot), B(anana), C(oconut) Smoothie

Most people only know apricots in their dried, prune-like form. In fact, fresh apricots in season are delicious. **SERVES 1**

½ cup (125 mL) water (or more, depending on preferred texture)

½ cup (125 mL) unsweetened coconut milk beverage

½ small frozen banana, chopped

½ cup (125 mL) sliced fresh apricots

¾ cup (175 mL) chopped cored unpeeled apple

1 serving unsweetened protein powder

2 teaspoons (10 mL) chia seeds

Ice cubes (optional)

Place ingredients in a blender in the order listed. Add ice if preferred. Blend until desired consistency is reached, adding more water to thin out if necessary.

---

## MODIFIED VERSION

For men or those 170 pounds (77 kg) and up, increase ingredients by one-third.

---

### Nutritional Information (per serving)

**Calories 329** • **Carbs 43 grams** • **Protein 26 grams** • **Fat 7 grams** • **Fiber 8 grams**

# Apple and Spice Cobbler Smoothie

When I was a kid in Toronto, my parents used to take me apple picking in the fall. We would come home with hundreds of apples (after a fun apple-throwing fight with my brothers), and my mother would make us homemade applesauce. This smoothie reminds me of that flavor.  **SERVES 1**

¼ cup (60 mL) water (or more, depending on preferred texture)

¾ cup (175 mL) unsweetened almond milk

1 cup (250 mL) chopped cored unpeeled apple

½ cup (125 mL) unsweetened applesauce

2 tablespoons (30 mL) ground flaxseed

1 serving unsweetened protein powder

¼ teaspoon (1 mL) cinnamon

Pinch of nutmeg

Ice cubes (optional)

Place ingredients in a blender in the order listed. Add ice if preferred. Blend until desired consistency is reached, adding more water to thin out if necessary.

---

### MODIFIED VERSION
For men or those 170 pounds (77 kg) and up, increase ingredients by one-third.

---

### Nutritional Information (per serving)

Calories 286  •  Carbs 32 grams  •  Protein 26 grams  •  Fat 8 grams  •  Fiber 9 grams

# Tropical Tofu Smoothie

Tofu is a great protein source in smoothies. It also has healthy fat and adds a nice creaminess.  **SERVES 1**

¼ cup (60 mL) unsweetened coconut milk beverage

¼ cup (60 mL) water (or more, depending on preferred texture)

½ cup (125 mL) chopped cored unpeeled apple

½ cup (125 mL) frozen chopped mango

½ kiwifruit, peeled and sliced

½ cup (125 mL) frozen chopped pineapple

2 tablespoons (30 mL) low-fat silken tofu

1½ teaspoons (7 mL) chia seeds

1 serving unsweetened protein powder

Zest and juice of 1 lime (optional)

4 ice cubes

Place ingredients in a blender in the order listed. Blend until desired consistency is reached, adding more water to thin out if necessary.

---

### MODIFIED VERSION
For men or those 170 pounds (77 kg) and up, increase ingredients by one-third.

---

**Nutritional Information (per serving)**

Calories 329  •  Carbs 45 grams  •  Protein 27 grams  •  Fat 6 grams  •  Fiber 8 grams

# Cantaloupe and Cucumber Smoothie

I call this my C and C smoothie. It has a very light texture and taste, but still manages to pack tons of protein and fiber, along with a touch of healthy fat.  **SERVES 1**

¼ cup (60 mL) water (or more, depending on preferred texture)

1 cup (250 mL) cubed cantaloupe

¾ cup (175 mL) chopped cored unpeeled apple

1 cup (250 mL) chopped unpeeled English cucumber

½ teaspoon (2 mL) grated fresh ginger

½ cup (125 mL) nonfat plain Greek yogurt

4 teaspoons (20 mL) chia seeds

Ice cubes (optional)

Place ingredients in a blender in the order listed. Add ice if preferred. Blend until desired consistency is reached, adding more water to thin out if necessary.

---

## MODIFIED VERSION

For men or those 170 pounds (77 kg) and up, increase ingredients by one-third.

---

### Nutritional Information (per serving)

Calories 272  •  Carbs 41 grams  •  Protein 19 grams  •  Fat 5 grams  •  Fiber 12 grams

# Creamy Spiced Pear Smoothie

Pears are a fall fruit. Shop then for the most delicious Bosc, Bartlett, or Anjou. The pumpkin spice adds a special flavor.   **SERVES 1**

¼ cup (60 mL) unsweetened almond milk

½ cup (125 mL) chopped cored unpeeled apple

¾ cup (175 mL) chopped cored unpeeled pear

5 almonds

½ cup (125 mL) nonfat plain Greek yogurt

½ serving unsweetened protein powder

½ teaspoon (2 mL) pumpkin pie spice

1 tablespoon (15 mL) chia seeds

Ice cubes (optional)

Place ingredients in a blender in the order listed. Add ice if preferred. Blend until desired consistency is reached, adding water to thin out if necessary.

---

### MODIFIED VERSION
For men or those 170 pounds (77 kg) and up, increase ingredients by one-third.

---

**Nutritional Information (per serving)**

Calories 317  •  Carbs 37 grams  •  Protein 26 grams  •  Fat 8 grams  •  Fiber 10 grams

# Banana Maple Nut Smoothie

Look for the darkest maple syrups. They are generally higher in nutrients and have much more maple flavor. **SERVES 1**

¼ cup (60 mL) unsweetened almond milk

1 medium frozen banana, chopped

2 dates, pitted

3 almonds

½ teaspoon (2 mL) pure maple syrup

4 teaspoons (20 mL) ground flaxseed

1 serving unsweetened protein powder

Ice cubes (optional)

Place ingredients in a blender in the order listed. Add ice if preferred. Blend until desired consistency is reached, adding water to thin out if necessary.

---

### MODIFIED VERSION

For men or those 170 pounds (77 kg) and up, increase ingredients by one-third.

---

**Nutritional Information (per serving)**

Calories 344 • Carbs 48 grams • Protein 27 grams • Fat 7 grams • Fiber 8 grams

# Apple Beet Smoothie

This smoothie has the most vibrant, amazing red color and is loaded with antioxidants.   **SERVES 1**

½ cup (125 mL) water (or more, depending on preferred texture)

1 cup (250 mL) chopped cored unpeeled apple

½ cup (125 mL) chopped raw beets

6 baby carrots

½ cup (125 mL) frozen chopped pineapple

1½ teaspoons (7 mL) ground flaxseed

1 serving unsweetened protein powder

Juice of 1 lemon (optional)

Ice cubes (optional)

Place ingredients in a blender in the order listed. Add ice if preferred. Blend until desired consistency is reached, adding more water to thin out if necessary.

---

## MODIFIED VERSION

For men or those 170 pounds (77 kg) and up, increase ingredients by one-third.

---

**Nutritional Information (per serving)**

Calories 284   •   **Carbs 41 grams**   •   **Protein 25 grams**   •   **Fat 4 grams**   •   **Fiber 8 grams**

# Power Breakfast Smoothie

Packed with 25 grams of protein and nearly 14 grams of fiber, this smoothie is super filling but with a low calorie cost.   **SERVES 1**

¼ cup (60 mL) water (or more, depending on preferred texture)

1 small frozen banana, chopped

¼ cup (60 mL) frozen blueberries

¼ cup (60 mL) fresh or frozen peaches

½ cup (125 mL) frozen raspberries

1 large orange, peeled and seeded

1 serving unsweetened protein powder

5 ice cubes

Place ingredients in a blender in the order listed. Blend until desired consistency is reached, adding more water to thin out if necessary.

---

### MODIFIED VERSION
For men or those 170 pounds (77 kg) and up, increase ingredients by one-third.

---

**Nutritional Information (per serving)**

Calories 324  •  Carbs 56 grams  •  Protein 25 grams  •  Fat 2 grams  •  Fiber 13 grams

# Cran-Berry Smoothie

Cranberries are loaded with phytonutrients and are a delicious addition to your diet. Look for unsweetened dried cranberries; many store-bought dried cranberries are loaded with added sugar and oil. **SERVES 1**

½ cup (125 mL) unsweetened dried cranberries, soaked in hot water for 5 minutes and drained

¾ cup (175 mL) frozen raspberries

1 ¼ cups (300 mL) frozen strawberries

1 tablespoon (15 mL) ground flaxseed

½ serving unsweetened protein powder

½ cup (125 mL) nonfat strawberry Greek yogurt

Ice cubes (optional)

Place ingredients in a blender in the order listed. Add ice if preferred. Blend until desired consistency is reached, adding water to thin out if necessary.

---

**MODIFIED VERSION**
For men or those 170 pounds (77 kg) and up, increase ingredients by one-third.

---

**Nutritional Information (per serving)**

Calories 320 • Carbs 48 grams • Protein 26 grams • Fat 4 grams • Fiber 18 grams

# Pomegranate Chia Smoothie

Pomegranate is one of the oldest fruits in the world. The edible seeds are a great source of fiber.

**SERVES 1**

½ cup (125 mL) water (or more, depending on preferred texture)

½ cup (125 mL) pomegranate seeds

½ cup (125 mL) frozen strawberries

½ cup (125 mL) frozen raspberries

½ medium frozen banana, chopped

1 tablespoon (15 mL) chia seeds

¾ cup (175 mL) nonfat plain Greek yogurt

Ice cubes (optional)

Place ingredients in a blender in the order listed. Add ice if preferred. Blend until desired consistency is reached, adding more water to thin out if necessary.

---

### MODIFIED VERSION
For men or those 170 pounds (77 kg) and up, increase ingredients by one-third.

---

**Nutritional Information (per serving)**

Calories 338 • Carbs 54 grams • Protein 22 grams • Fat 6 grams • Fiber 14 grams

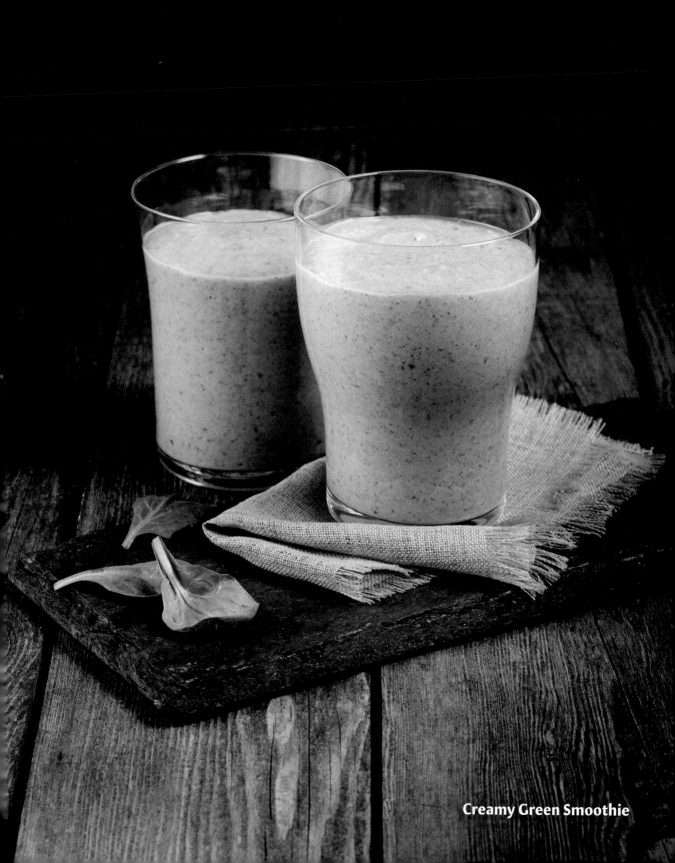

Creamy Green Smoothie

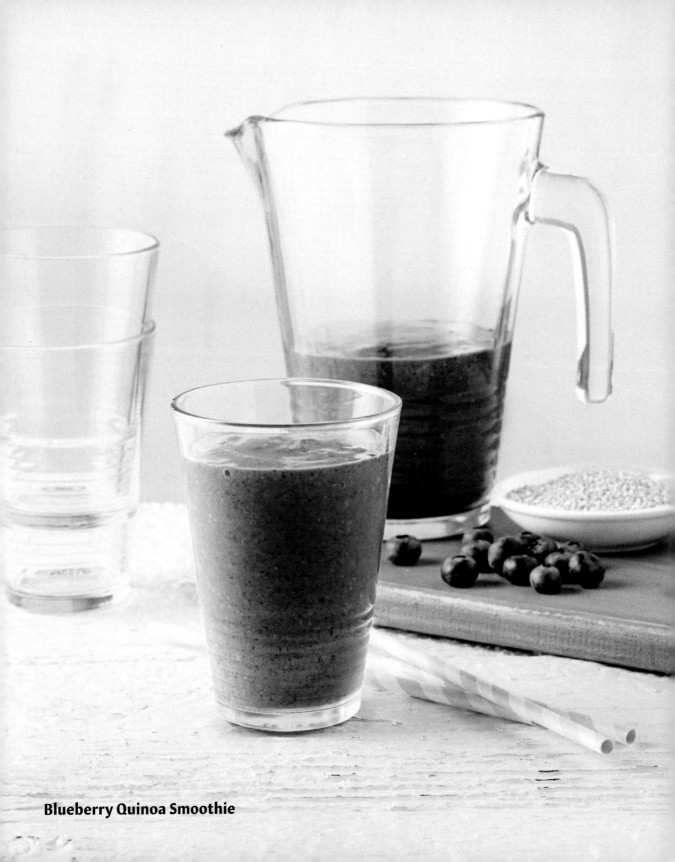

**Blueberry Quinoa Smoothie**

Carrot Pineapple Cake Smoothie

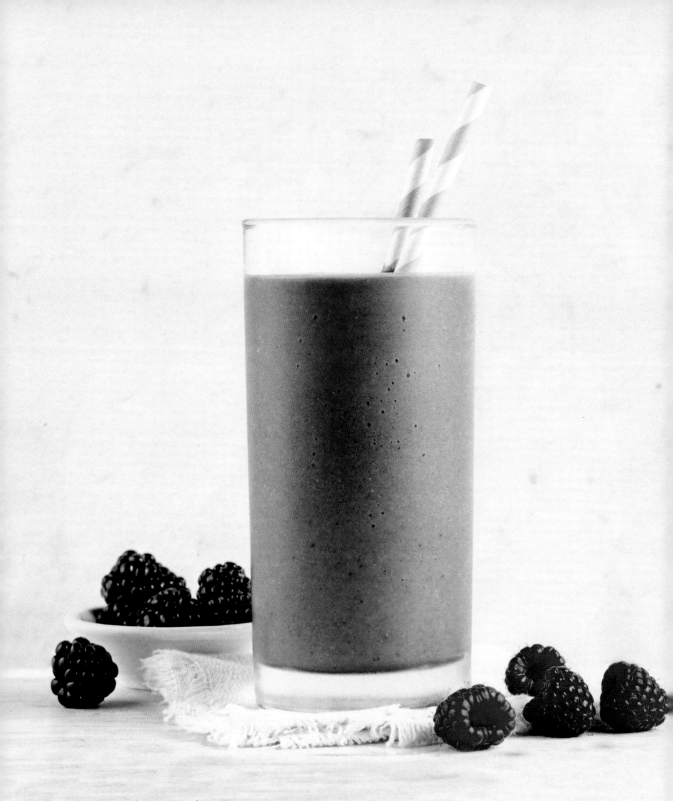

**Purple Popsicle Smoothie**

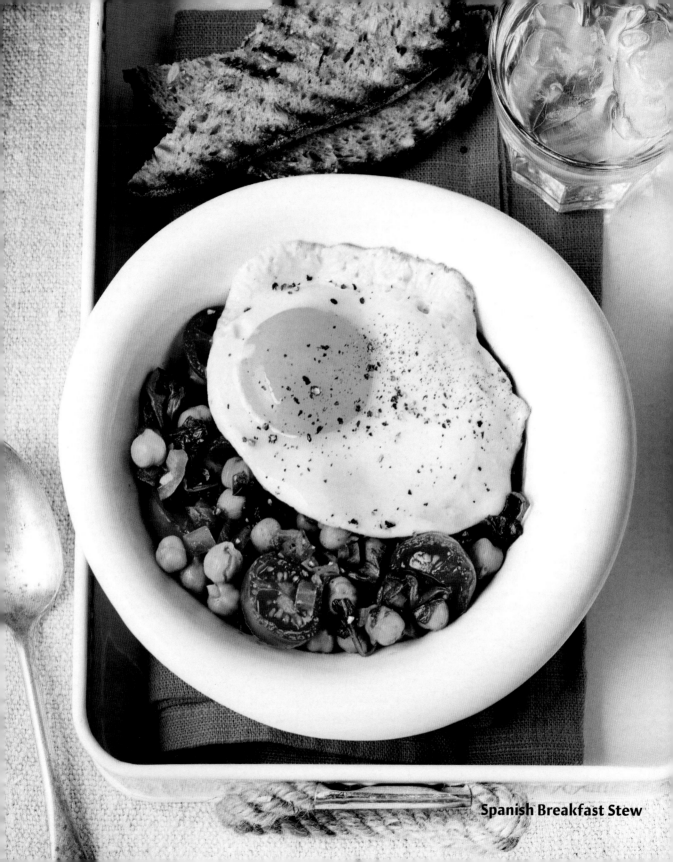

Spanish Breakfast Stew

Asian Chicken Salad

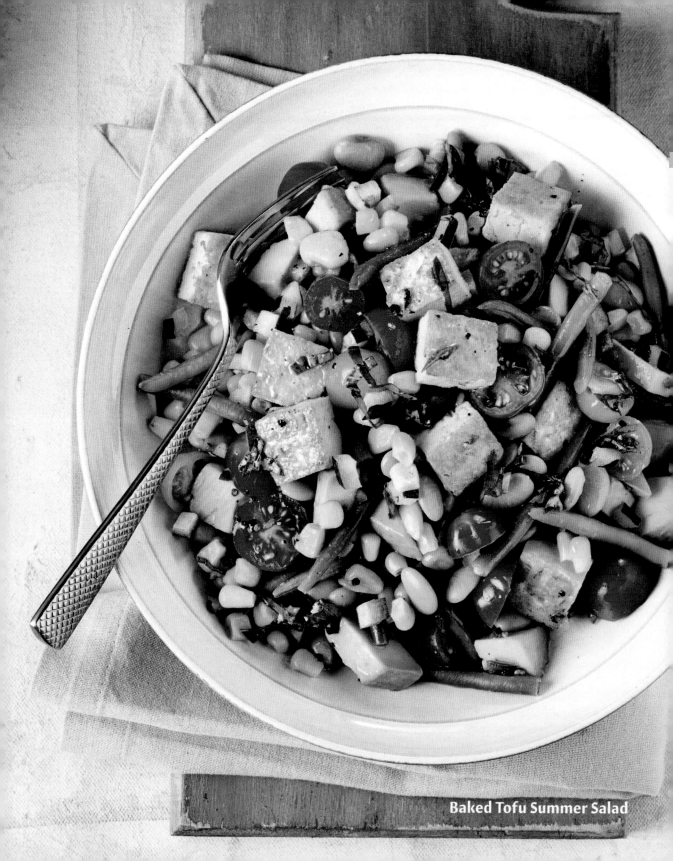

Baked Tofu Summer Salad

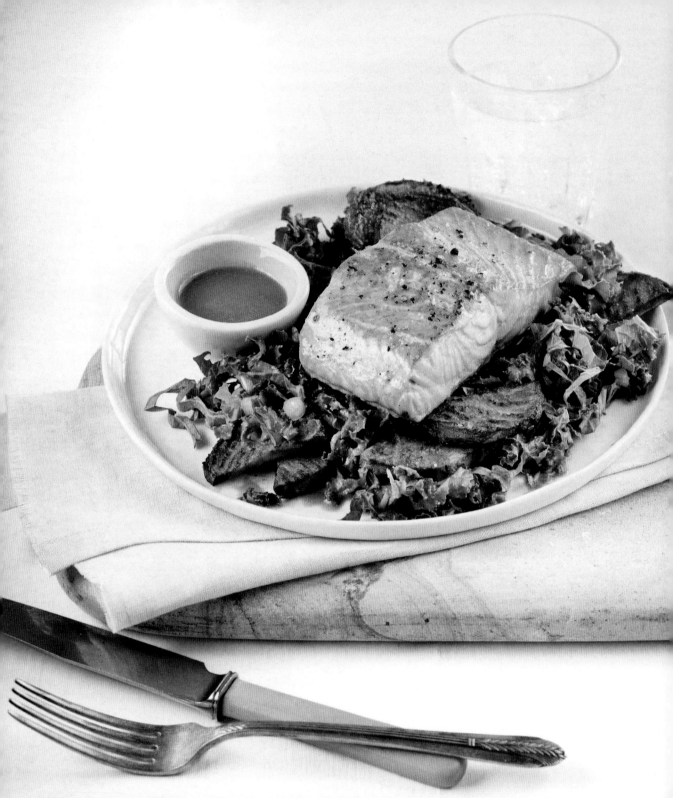

**Salmon, Kale, and Roasted Sweet Potato Salad with Miso Vinaigrette**

# Energy Booster Smoothie

I learned to love dates when I was working in Istanbul. They are an amazing natural sweetener.

**SERVES 1**

½ cup (125 mL) water (or more, depending on preferred texture)

¾ cup (175 mL) frozen raspberries

2 dates, pitted

1 cup (250 mL) frozen chopped mango

¾ cup (175 mL) nonfat plain Greek yogurt

Juice of 1 lime (optional)

4 ice cubes

Place ingredients in a blender in the order listed. Blend until desired consistency is reached, adding more water to thin out if necessary.

---

## MODIFIED VERSION

For men or those 170 pounds (77 kg) and up, increase ingredients by one-third.

---

### Nutritional Information (per serving)

Calories 299 • Carbs 58 grams • Protein 20 grams • Fat 1 grams • Fiber 11 grams

# Blackberry Grape Smoothie

This smoothie tastes (and looks) an awful lot like cotton candy. But it's so much healthier! **SERVES 1**

½ cup (125 mL) water (or more, depending on preferred texture)

½ cup (125 mL) unsweetened coconut milk beverage

1 cup (250 mL) chopped cored unpeeled apple

½ small frozen banana, chopped

½ cup (125 mL) frozen raspberries

½ cup (125 mL) frozen red grapes

½ cup (125 mL) frozen blackberries

1 serving unsweetened protein powder

4 ice cubes

Place ingredients in a blender in the order listed. Blend until desired consistency is reached, adding more water to thin out if necessary.

---

### MODIFIED VERSION
For men or those 170 pounds (77 kg) and up, increase ingredients by one-third.

---

**Nutritional Information (per serving)**

Calories 346 • Carbs 54 grams • Protein 25 grams • Fat 5 grams • Fiber 9 grams

# Creamy Avocado Berry Smoothie

I love the creamy texture of this smoothie. If you're not a kale enthusiast, don't worry—the taste is entirely hidden by the sweetness of the raspberries and banana.   **SERVES 1**

½ cup (125 mL) water (or more, depending on preferred texture)

¼ avocado, peeled and sliced

1 cup (250 mL) frozen raspberries

½ small frozen banana, chopped

½ cup (125 mL) nonfat plain Greek yogurt

½ cup (125 mL) chopped kale

½ serving unsweetened protein powder

4 ice cubes

Place ingredients in a blender in the order listed. Blend until desired consistency is reached, adding more water to thin out if necessary.

---

### MODIFIED VERSION
For men or those 170 pounds (77 kg) and up, increase ingredients by one-third.

---

**Nutritional Information (per serving)**

Calories 316  •  Carbs 39 grams  •  Protein 26 grams  •  Fat 8 grams  •  Fiber 14 grams

# Coco-Berry Smoothie

This smoothie contains my top three favorite fiber-rich fruits: apple, strawberries, and raspberries.

**SERVES 1**

½ cup (125 mL) coconut water

½ cup (125 mL) frozen strawberries

¾ cup (175 mL) frozen raspberries

1 cup (250 mL) chopped cored unpeeled apple

½ small frozen banana, chopped

¾ serving unsweetened protein powder

4 ice cubes (optional)

Place ingredients in a blender in the order listed. Blend until desired consistency is reached, adding water to thin out if necessary.

---

### MODIFIED VERSION

For men or those 170 pounds (77 kg) and up, increase ingredients by one-third.

---

**Nutritional Information (per serving)**

Calories 270 • Carbs 50 grams • Protein 19 grams • Fat 2 grams • Fiber 11 grams

# Pineapple Kale Smoothie

I fell in love with pineapple when I spent a year working in Oahu, Hawaii. Here, the sweetness of the pineapple balances the bitterness of the kale and the heat of the ginger. **SERVES 1**

1 cup (250 mL) water (or more, depending on preferred texture)

1 cup (250 mL) chopped cored unpeeled apple

2 cups (500 mL) chopped kale

¾ teaspoon (4 mL) grated fresh ginger

¾ cup (175 mL) frozen chopped pineapple

1 serving unsweetened protein powder

Juice of 1 lemon (optional)

Ice cubes (optional)

Place ingredients in a blender in the order listed. Add ice if preferred. Blend until desired consistency is reached, adding more water to thin out if necessary.

---

**MODIFIED VERSION**

For men or those 170 pounds (77 kg) and up, increase ingredients by one-third.

---

**Nutritional Information (per serving)**

Calories 318 • Carbs 54 grams • Protein 28 grams • Fat 3 grams • Fiber 10 grams

# Avocado Banana Smoothie

This smoothie is teeming with vitamin C, and the avocado and banana give it an amazing creamy consistency. **SERVES 1**

¼ cup (60 mL) water (or more, depending on preferred texture)

½ small frozen banana, chopped

½ cup (125 mL) chopped cored unpeeled apple

¼ avocado, peeled and sliced

½ small orange, peeled and seeded

½ serving unsweetened protein powder

⅓ cup (75 mL) nonfat plain Greek yogurt

Ice cubes (optional)

Place ingredients in a blender in the order listed. Add ice if preferred. Blend until desired consistency is reached, adding more water to thin out if necessary.

---

### MODIFIED VERSION
For men or those 170 pounds (77 kg) and up, increase ingredients by one-third.

---

**Nutritional Information (per serving)**

Calories 292 • Carbs 38 grams • Protein 22 grams • Fat 7 grams • Fiber 10 grams

# Creamy Green Smoothie

This smoothie contains two amazing sources of essential fatty acids: chia seeds and avocado. **SERVES 1**

½ cup (125 mL) water (or more, depending on preferred texture)

½ small frozen banana, chopped

2½ cups (625 mL) fresh spinach

½ cup (125 mL) chopped cored unpeeled apple

⅛ avocado, peeled and sliced

½ serving unsweetened protein powder

1 tablespoon (15 mL) chia seeds

½ cup (125 mL) nonfat plain Greek yogurt

Ice cubes (optional)

Place ingredients in a blender in the order listed. Add ice if preferred. Blend until desired consistency is reached, adding more water to thin out if necessary.

---

**MODIFIED VERSION**
For men or those 170 pounds (77 kg) and up, increase ingredients by one-third.

---

**Nutritional Information (per serving)**

Calories 299 • Carbs 34 grams • Protein 26 grams • Fat 8 grams • Fiber 10 grams

# Minty Melon Smoothie

This refreshing smoothie was inspired by an amazing watermelon and mint salad I had at one of my friend José Andrés's restaurants.  **SERVES 1**

½ large unpeeled English cucumber, chopped

½ cup (125 mL) chopped cored unpeeled apple

1⅓ cups (325 mL) chopped honeydew melon

1½ teaspoons (7 mL) chopped fresh mint

1 serving unsweetened protein powder

1 tablespoon (15 mL) chia seeds

Juice of ½ lime (optional)

Ice cubes (optional)

Place ingredients in a blender in the order listed. Add ice if preferred. Blend until desired consistency is reached, adding water to thin out if necessary.

---

### MODIFIED VERSION

For men or those 170 pounds (77 kg) and up, increase ingredients by one-third.

---

**Nutritional Information (per serving)**

Calories 298  •  Carbs 42 grams  •  Protein 23 grams  •  Fat 6 grams  •  Fiber 9 grams

# Spinach, Apple, and Carrot Smoothie

Spinach and apple are a great combination. I added carrot to this smoothie to give it a natural sweetness and a delightful texture. **SERVES 1**

½ cup (125 mL) water (or more, depending on preferred texture)

1 cup (250 mL) chopped cored unpeeled apple

5 baby carrots

1 serving unsweetened protein powder

½ medium orange, peeled and seeded

2½ cups (625 mL) fresh spinach

¾ teaspoon (4 mL) grated fresh ginger

Juice of 1 lemon (optional)

Ice cubes (optional)

Place ingredients in a blender in the order listed. Add ice if preferred. Blend until desired consistency is reached, adding more water to thin out if necessary.

---

### MODIFIED VERSION
For men or those 170 pounds (77 kg) and up, increase ingredients by one-third.

---

**Nutritional Information (per serving)**

Calories 294 • Carbs 49 grams • Protein 26 grams • Fat 2 grams • Fiber 11 grams

# Spinach Kiwi Smoothie

I love kiwis! They're one of the few fruits whose seeds you can actually eat. In fact, go ahead and eat the skin too (just brush off the fine hairs beforehand).   **SERVES 1**

½ cup (125 mL) water (or more, depending on preferred texture)

2 kiwifruit, peeled and chopped

2½ cups (625 mL) fresh spinach

1 small frozen banana, chopped

4 almonds

½ cup (125 mL) nonfat plain Greek yogurt

Ice cubes (optional)

Place ingredients in a blender in the order listed. Add ice if preferred. Blend until desired consistency is reached, adding more water to thin out if necessary.

---

### MODIFIED VERSION
For men or those 170 pounds (77 kg) and up, increase ingredients by one-third.

---

### Nutritional Information (per serving)

Calories 311  •  Carbs 58 grams  •  Protein 18 grams  •  Fat 4 grams  •  Fiber 11 grams

# Spinach and Peach Smoothie

This smoothie is dedicated to all my friends who live in Georgia. Fresh peaches are amazing when—and only when—they're in season. Otherwise, stick to frozen.   **SERVES 1**

½ cup (125 mL) unsweetened almond milk

1½ cups (375 mL) fresh or frozen sliced peaches

8 almonds

½ serving unsweetened protein powder

½ teaspoon (2 mL) grated fresh ginger

2½ cups (625 mL) fresh spinach

Ice cubes (optional)

Place ingredients in a blender in the order listed. Add ice if preferred. Blend until desired consistency is reached, adding water to thin out if necessary.

---

### MODIFIED VERSION
For men or those 170 pounds (77 kg) and up, increase ingredients by one-third.

---

**Nutritional Information (per serving)**

Calories 272  •  Carbs 40 grams  •  Protein 18 grams  •  Fat 8 grams  •  Fiber 9 grams

# Coconut Spinach Smoothie

Coconut water is loaded with potassium and adds a gentle sweetness and coconut flavor.   **SERVES 1**

½ cup (125 mL) coconut water

1 cup (250 mL) seedless green or red grapes

1 small frozen banana, chopped

2½ cups (625 mL) fresh spinach

½ serving unsweetened protein powder

1 tablespoon (15 mL) chia seeds

Ice cubes (optional)

Place ingredients in a blender in the order listed. Add ice if preferred. Blend until desired consistency is reached, adding water to thin out if necessary.

---

**MODIFIED VERSION**

For men or those 170 pounds (77 kg) and up, increase ingredients by one-third.

---

**Nutritional Information (per serving)**

Calories 288  •  Carbs 49 grams  •  Protein 18 grams  •  Fat 6 grams  •  Fiber 10 grams

# Nutty Kale Berry Smoothie

I love this smoothie when I'm hungry. The healthy fats in the almonds and flaxseeds make it really filling.

**SERVES 1**

½ cup (125 mL) unsweetened almond milk

2 cups (500 mL) chopped kale

1 small frozen banana, chopped

½ cup (125 mL) frozen raspberries

4 almonds

1 tablespoon (15 mL) ground flaxseed

½ serving unsweetened protein powder

Ice cubes (optional)

Place ingredients in a blender in the order listed. Add ice if preferred. Blend until desired consistency is reached, adding water to thin out if necessary.

---

### MODIFIED VERSION
For men or those 170 pounds (77 kg) and up, increase ingredients by one-third.

---

**Nutritional Information (per serving)**

Calories 341 • Carbs 53 grams • Protein 21 grams • Fat 8 grams • Fiber 15 grams

# Watermelon Orange Smoothie

You'll never notice the spinach hidden in this smoothie. Great for kids—and even grown-ups—who won't eat their veggies.  **SERVES 1**

¾ cup (175 mL) water (or more, depending on preferred texture)

½ medium orange, peeled and seeded

2½ cups (625 mL) fresh spinach

1½ cups (375 mL) chopped seeded watermelon

¼ large unpeeled English cucumber, chopped

1 serving unsweetened protein powder

Juice of 1 lemon (optional)

Ice cubes (optional)

Place ingredients in a blender in the order listed. Add ice if preferred. Blend until desired consistency is reached, adding more water to thin out if necessary.

---

### MODIFIED VERSION
For men or those 170 pounds (77 kg) and up, increase ingredients by one-third.

---

**Nutritional Information (per serving)**

Calories 302 • Carbs 48 grams • Protein 28 grams • Fat 3 grams • Fiber 9 grams

# Mango Lime Yogurt Smoothie

I got the idea for this smoothie when I was working in Singapore. On just about every street corner you can buy sliced mangoes with lime juice and chili powder.   **SERVES 1**

1/8 avocado, peeled and sliced

3/4 cup (175 mL) chopped cored unpeeled apple

3/4 cup (175 mL) frozen chopped mango

1/2 cup (125 mL) nonfat plain Greek yogurt

1/2 serving unsweetened protein powder

1 tablespoon (15 mL) ground flaxseed

Chili powder to taste (optional)

Juice of 1 lime (optional)

Ice cubes (optional)

Place ingredients in a blender in the order listed. Add ice if preferred. Blend until desired consistency is reached, adding water to thin out if necessary.

---

### MODIFIED VERSION
For men or those 170 pounds (77 kg) and up, increase ingredients by one-third.

---

**Nutritional Information (per serving)**

Calories 309  •  Carbs 42 grams  •  Protein 25 grams  •  Fat 7 grams  •  Fiber 8 grams

# Apple Jack Smoothie

This smoothie is incredibly hydrating. The cucumber gives it a crisp and clean flavor.  **SERVES 1**

¼ cup (60 mL) water (or more, depending on preferred texture)

¾ cup (175 mL) unsweetened coconut milk beverage

1 cup (250 mL) chopped cored unpeeled apple

½ large unpeeled English cucumber, chopped

½ small frozen banana, chopped

1 teaspoon (5 mL) grated fresh ginger

2 teaspoons (10 mL) chia seeds

¾ serving unsweetened protein powder

¼ teaspoon (1 mL) cinnamon

Ice cubes (optional)

Place ingredients in a blender in the order listed. Add ice if preferred. Blend until desired consistency is reached, adding more water to thin out if necessary.

---

### MODIFIED VERSION
For men or those 170 pounds (77 kg) and up, increase ingredients by one-third.

---

**Nutritional Information (per serving)**

Calories 299  •  Carbs 40 grams  •  Protein 21 grams  •  Fat 8 grams  •  Fiber 9 grams

# Hippy Hippy Shake

There are 13 grams of fiber hiding in this smoothie. That's nearly half of your daily fiber needs.

**SERVES 1**

½ cup (125 mL) water (or more, depending on preferred texture)

2½ cups (625 mL) fresh spinach

½ cup (125 mL) chopped cored unpeeled apple

2 cups (500 mL) chopped kale

1 cup (250 mL) frozen chopped pineapple

1 tablespoon (15 mL) ground flaxseed

½ serving unsweetened protein powder

Ice cubes (optional)

Place ingredients in a blender in the order listed. Add ice if preferred. Blend until desired consistency is reached, adding more water to thin out if necessary.

---

## MODIFIED VERSION

For men or those 170 pounds (77 kg) and up, increase ingredients by one-third.

---

**Nutritional Information (per serving)**

Calories 284 • Carbs 47 grams • Protein 18 grams • Fat 5 grams • Fiber 13 grams

# Mango Coconut Smoothie

Loaded with sweet tropical flavors, this smoothie has tons of omega fatty acids.   **SERVES 1**

½ cup (125 mL) water (or more, depending on preferred texture)

½ small frozen banana, chopped

¾ cup (175 mL) frozen chopped mango

¼ cup (60 mL) unsweetened shredded coconut

½ serving unsweetened protein powder

4 teaspoons (20 mL) chia seeds

¼ cup (60 mL) nonfat plain Greek yogurt

Ice cubes (optional)

Place ingredients in a blender in the order listed. Add ice if preferred. Blend until desired consistency is reached, adding more water to thin out if necessary.

---

### MODIFIED VERSION
For men or those 170 pounds (77 kg) and up, increase ingredients by one-third.

---

### Nutritional Information (per serving)

Calories 301  •  Carbs 43 grams  •  Protein 21 grams  •  Fat 8 grams  •  Fiber 9 grams

# Immunity Boost Smoothie

Hard to believe this smoothie is only 300 calories—it tastes like sorbet.  **SERVES 1**

½ cup (125 mL) water (or more, depending on preferred texture)

½ cup (125 mL) unsweetened almond milk

½ cup (125 mL) frozen chopped mango

½ cup (125 mL) chopped cantaloupe

½ cup (125 mL) frozen chopped pineapple

1 tablespoon (15 mL) chia seeds

1 serving unsweetened protein powder

5 ice cubes

Place ingredients in a blender in the order listed. Blend until desired consistency is reached, adding more water to thin out if necessary.

---

**MODIFIED VERSION**

For men or those 170 pounds (77 kg) and up, increase ingredients by one-third.

---

**Nutritional Information (per serving)**

**Calories 310  •  Carbs 38 grams  •  Protein 26 grams  •  Fat 8 grams  •  Fiber 8 grams**

# Pineapple Cooler Smoothie

Imagine yourself on a beach bathing in sunshine, drinking this smoothie.  **SERVES 1**

½ cup (125 mL) water (or more, depending on preferred texture)

½ cup (125 mL) unsweetened coconut milk beverage

1 cup (250 mL) frozen chopped pineapple

1 cup (250 mL) chopped cored unpeeled apple

½ serving unsweetened protein powder

½ cup (125 mL) nonfat plain Greek yogurt

2 teaspoons (10 mL) chia seeds

4 ice cubes

Place ingredients in a blender in the order listed. Blend until desired consistency is reached, adding more water to thin out if necessary.

---

### MODIFIED VERSION

For men or those 170 pounds (77 kg) and up, increase ingredients by one-third.

---

**Nutritional Information (per serving)**

Calories 334  •  Carbs 49 grams  •  Protein 24 grams  •  Fat 7 grams  •  Fiber 8 grams

# Pumpkin Spice Smoothie

Pumpkin is loaded with vitamin A and fiber. I love this smoothie in the fall.  **SERVES 1**

¼ cup (60 mL) low-fat cottage cheese

¼ cup (60 mL) unsweetened pumpkin purée

4 almonds

½ cup (125 mL) water (or more, depending on preferred texture)

1½ cups (375 mL) chopped cored unpeeled apple

¾ cup (175 mL) unsweetened almond milk

1 tablespoon (15 mL) ground flaxseed

½ teaspoon (2 mL) pumpkin pie spice

½ serving unsweetened protein powder

Ice cubes (optional)

1. Place cottage cheese, pumpkin purée, and almonds in a blender. Blend until smooth, adding small amounts of water as needed.
2. Add remaining ingredients. Add ice if preferred. Blend until desired consistency is reached, adding more water to thin out if necessary.

---

### MODIFIED VERSION
For men or those 170 pounds (77 kg) and up, increase ingredients by one-third.

---

**Nutritional Information (per serving)**

Calories 296  •  Carbs 39 grams  •  Protein 23 grams  •  Fat 8 grams  •  Fiber 10 grams

# Orange Creamsicle Smoothie

After many failed attempts, I finally perfected this creamsicle smoothie. It has that amazing creamy orange flavor.   **SERVES 1**

½ cup (125 mL) unsweetened coconut milk beverage

1 large orange, peeled and seeded

½ medium frozen banana, chopped

½ serving unsweetened protein powder

½ cup (125 mL) nonfat plain Greek yogurt

1½ teaspoons (7 mL) chia seeds

½ teaspoon (2 mL) vanilla extract (optional)

4 ice cubes

Place ingredients in a blender in the order listed. Blend until desired consistency is reached, adding water to thin out if necessary.

---

**MODIFIED VERSION**

For men or those 170 pounds (77 kg) and up, increase ingredients by one-third.

---

**Nutritional Information (per serving)**

Calories 356  •  Carbs 52 grams  •  Protein 25 grams  •  Fat 5 grams  •  Fiber 13 grams

# Carrot Pineapple Cake Smoothie

This smoothie gets its fiber from multiple sources, and it keeps you satisfied until your next meal.
**SERVES 1**

¾ cup (175 mL) unsweetened almond milk

7 baby carrots

1 cup (250 mL) frozen chopped pineapple

½ cup (125 mL) chopped cored unpeeled apple

1 tablespoon (15 mL) ground flaxseed

½ teaspoon (2 mL) grated fresh ginger

1 serving unsweetened protein powder

Ice cubes (optional)

Place ingredients in a blender in the order listed. Add ice if preferred. Blend until desired consistency is reached, adding water to thin out if necessary.

---

**MODIFIED VERSION**
For men or those 170 pounds (77 kg) and up, increase ingredients by one-third.

---

**Nutritional Information (per serving)**

**Calories 305 • Carbs 41 grams • Protein 26 grams • Fat 6 grams • Fiber 8 grams**

# Almond Apple Berry Smoothie

I use almond milk in this smoothie, but you can boost the protein if you use skim milk or soy milk.

**SERVES 1**

¾ cup (175 mL) unsweetened almond milk

½ cup (125 mL) chopped cored unpeeled apple

½ small frozen banana, chopped

½ cup (125 mL) frozen strawberries

½ cup (125 mL) frozen blueberries

½ serving unsweetened protein powder

1½ teaspoons (7 mL) chia seeds

½ cup (125 mL) nonfat plain Greek yogurt

Ice cubes (optional)

Place ingredients in a blender in the order listed. Add ice if preferred. Blend until desired consistency is reached, adding water to thin out if necessary.

---

### MODIFIED VERSION
For men or those 170 pounds (77 kg) and up, increase ingredients by one-third.

---

**Nutritional Information (per serving)**

Calories 311 • Carbs 45 grams • Protein 24 grams • Fat 6 grams • Fiber 9 grams

# Purple Popsicle Smoothie

The blackberry and raspberry combination gives this smoothie its vibrant red-purple color and its whopping 16 grams of fiber.  **SERVES** 1

½ cup (125 mL) water (or more, depending on preferred texture)

½ cup (125 mL) unsweetened coconut milk beverage

¼ cup (60 mL) fresh or frozen blackberries

1 cup (250 mL) frozen raspberries

½ cup (125 mL) frozen chopped mango

½ small orange, peeled and seeded

1 serving unsweetened protein powder

Ice cubes (optional)

Place ingredients in a blender in the order listed. Add ice if preferred. Blend until desired consistency is reached, adding more water to thin out if necessary.

---

### MODIFIED VERSION
For men or those 170 pounds (77 kg) and up, increase ingredients by one-third.

---

**Nutritional Information (per serving)**

Calories 318  •  Carbs 49 grams  •  Protein 25 grams  •  Fat 5 grams  •  Fiber 16 grams

# Avocado Blueberry Smoothie

This is one of my favorite smoothies. It looks so good, you can taste it before you put it to your lips. I can't taste the kale at all.   **SERVES 1**

¾ cup (175 mL) water (or more, depending on preferred texture)

1 small orange, peeled and seeded

½ cup (125 mL) chopped kale

½ cup (125 mL) frozen blueberries

½ small frozen banana, chopped

¼ avocado, peeled and sliced

¾ serving unsweetened protein powder

Ice cubes (optional)

Place ingredients in a blender in the order listed. Add ice if preferred. Blend until desired consistency is reached, adding more water to thin out if necessary.

---

### MODIFIED VERSION
For men or those 170 pounds (77 kg) and up, increase ingredients by one-third.

---

**Nutritional Information (per serving)**

Calories 327  •  Carbs 48 grams  •  Protein 21 grams  •  Fat 8 grams  •  Fiber 13 grams

# Antioxidant Smoothie

This smoothie is packed with antioxidants. Generally speaking, the brighter the natural color, the healthier something is for you.   **SERVES 1**

¾ cup (175 mL) water (or more, depending on preferred texture)

½ cup (125 mL) frozen blueberries

½ cup (125 mL) frozen pitted cherries

½ cup (125 mL) frozen strawberries

½ cup (125 mL) frozen raspberries

⅛ avocado, peeled and sliced

½ cup (125 mL) nonfat plain Greek yogurt

½ serving unsweetened protein powder

4 ice cubes

Place ingredients in a blender in the order listed. Blend until desired consistency is reached, adding more water to thin out if necessary.

---

### MODIFIED VERSION
For men or those 170 pounds (77 kg) and up, increase ingredients by one-third.

---

**Nutritional Information (per serving)**

Calories 297   •   Carbs 42 grams   •   Protein 25 grams   •   Fat 5 grams   •   Fiber 11 grams

# Blueberry and Maple Oat Smoothie

An ode to my Canadian roots, this smoothie has a subtle maple flavor. Recent research has shown that maple syrup is high in certain antioxidants.  **SERVES 1**

¼ cup (60 mL) rolled oats

½ cup (125 mL) nonfat plain Greek yogurt

½ cup (125 mL) unsweetened almond milk

¼ cup (60 mL) frozen blueberries

½ cup (125 mL) frozen raspberries

1 cup (250 mL) chopped cored unpeeled apple

¼ serving unsweetened protein powder

1 tablespoon (15 mL) ground flaxseed

¾ teaspoon (4 mL) pure maple syrup

Ice cubes (optional)

1. Stir together oats and yogurt. Cover and let sit in the fridge overnight.
2. Put oats and remaining ingredients in a blender in the order listed. Add ice if preferred. Blend until desired consistency is reached, adding water to thin out if necessary.

---

**MODIFIED VERSION**

For men or those 170 pounds (77 kg) and up, increase ingredients by one-third.

---

**Nutritional Information (per serving)**

Calories 328 • Carbs 53 grams • Protein 21 grams • Fat 6 grams • Fiber 13 grams

# Nuts and Berry Breakfast Smoothie

I opted for pistachios to boost the healthy fat, fiber, and protein content of this smoothie. They also add lots of flavor. Make sure to buy unroasted, unsalted pistachios in the shell and separate them yourself. Roasting chemically changes the composition of nuts, often increasing saturated fat and decreasing overall health benefits. **SERVES 1**

½ cup (125 mL) unsweetened almond milk

½ cup (125 mL) frozen blueberries

½ small frozen banana, chopped

½ cup (125 mL) chopped cored unpeeled pear

1 cup (250 mL) frozen strawberries

6 pistachios

1 serving unsweetened protein powder

1½ teaspoons (7 mL) ground flaxseed

Ice cubes (optional)

Place ingredients in a blender in the order listed. Add ice if preferred. Blend until desired consistency is reached, adding water to thin out if necessary.

---

### MODIFIED VERSION
For men or those 170 pounds (77 kg) and up, increase ingredients by one-third.

---

**Nutritional Information (per serving)**

Calories 337  •  Carbs 49 grams  •  Protein 26 grams  •  Fat 6 grams  •  Fiber 11 grams

# Blueberry Quinoa Smoothie

Quinoa, the Peruvian super-grain, is nearly a complete food in and of itself. It's a complete protein (meaning it provides all the essential amino acids), it's high in water-soluble fiber, and it contains healthy fats.
**SERVES 1**

2 tablespoons (30 mL) cooked quinoa (preferably white)

1 cup (250 mL) unsweetened almond milk

½ large frozen banana, chopped

½ cup (125 mL) frozen raspberries

¾ cup (175 mL) frozen blueberries

½ serving unsweetened protein powder

1 tablespoon (15 mL) wheat germ

Ice cubes (optional)

Place all ingredients in a blender in the order listed. Add ice if preferred. Blend until desired consistency is reached, adding water to thin out if necessary.

---

### MODIFIED VERSION
For men or those 170 pounds (77 kg) and up, increase ingredients by one-third.

---

**Nutritional Information (per serving)**

Calories 307 • Carbs 52 grams • Protein 17 grams • Fat 6 grams • Fiber 12 grams

# Cocoa Banana Peanut Butter (CBPB) Smoothie

Can you say "too good to be healthy"?   **SERVES 1**

1½ cups (375 mL) unsweetened almond milk

1 large frozen banana, chopped

2 dates, pitted

2 tablespoons (30 mL) powdered peanut butter
   (or 1½ teaspoons/7 mL reduced-fat peanut butter, or 5 peanuts)

½ serving unsweetened protein powder

1½ teaspoons (7 mL) unsweetened cocoa powder

4 ice cubes

Place ingredients in a blender in the order listed. Blend until desired consistency is reached, adding water to thin out if necessary.

---

**MODIFIED VERSION**

For men or those 170 pounds (77 kg) and up, increase ingredients by one-third.

---

**Nutritional Information (per serving)**

**Calories 320  •  Carbs 53 grams  •  Protein 19 grams  •  Fat 7 grams  •  Fiber 8 grams**

# Banana Prune Smoothie

The prunes give this smoothie tons of added fiber and the perfect hint of sweetness.   SERVES 1

½ cup (125 mL) unsweetened almond milk

1 small frozen banana, chopped

2 pitted dried prunes, soaked in hot water for 5 minutes and drained

1 serving unsweetened protein powder

2 tablespoons (30 mL) ground flaxseed

4 ice cubes

Place ingredients in a blender in the order listed. Blend until desired consistency is reached, adding water to thin out if necessary.

---

### MODIFIED VERSION
For men or those 170 pounds (77 kg) and up, increase ingredients by one-third.

---

**Nutritional Information (per serving)**

Calories 325 • Carbs 43 grams • Protein 27 grams • Fat 7 grams • Fiber 9 grams

# Date Smoothie

I came up with this shake when I was working in the Middle East. Everyone kept offering me delicious dates as a snack, so I started adding them to my smoothies. Yum!   **SERVES 1**

½ cup (125 mL) unsweetened coconut milk beverage

1 small frozen banana, chopped

3 Medjool dates, pitted, soaked in hot water for 5 minutes and drained

½ serving unsweetened protein powder

2 teaspoons (10 mL) chia seeds

¼ cup (60 mL) nonfat plain Greek yogurt

3 almonds

4 ice cubes

Place ingredients in a blender in the order listed. Blend until desired consistency is reached, adding water to thin out if necessary.

---

### MODIFIED VERSION
For men or those 170 pounds (77 kg) and up, increase ingredients by one-third.

---

**Nutritional Information (per serving)**

Calories 348  •  Carbs 53 grams  •  Protein 20 grams  •  Fat 8 grams  •  Fiber 8 grams

# Coconut Ginger Carrot Smoothie

Like liquid carrot cake! Sweet and savory.   **SERVES 1**

¾ cup (175 mL) unsweetened coconut milk beverage

1 cup (250 mL) sliced cored unpeeled pears

6 baby carrots

1 serving unsweetened protein powder

2 teaspoons (10 mL) chia seeds

½ teaspoon (2 mL) grated fresh ginger

Ice cubes (optional)

Place ingredients in a blender in the order listed. Add ice if preferred. Blend until desired consistency is reached, adding water to thin out if necessary.

---

### MODIFIED VERSION

For men or those 170 pounds (77 kg) and up, increase ingredients by one-third.

---

**Nutritional Information (per serving)**

Calories 316 • Carbs 37 grams • Protein 25 grams • Fat 8 grams • Fiber 9 grams

# Energizing Chai Tea Smoothie

This has got to be the perfect breakfast smoothie. **SERVES 1**

1 cup (250 mL) brewed chai tea, cooled

1 small frozen banana, chopped

¾ cup (175 mL) chopped cored unpeeled apple

8 almonds

¼ teaspoon (1 mL) cinnamon

1½ teaspoons (7 mL) chia seeds

¾ serving unsweetened protein powder

Ice cubes (optional)

Place ingredients in a blender in the order listed. Add ice if preferred. Blend until desired consistency is reached, adding water to thin out if necessary.

---

**MODIFIED VERSION**

For men or those 170 pounds (77 kg) and up, increase ingredients by one-third.

---

**Nutritional Information (per serving)**

Calories 336 • Carbs 44 grams • Protein 26 grams • Fat 8 grams • Fiber 8 grams

# Candied Almond Smoothie

Those of you who are chocoholics (like me) will love the hit of cocoa in this smoothie.   SERVES 1

¾ cup (175 mL) unsweetened almond milk

1 small frozen banana, chopped

1½ teaspoons (7 mL) unsweetened cocoa powder

½ serving unsweetened protein powder

1 tablespoon (15 mL) ground flaxseed

5 almonds

3 dates, pitted

5 ice cubes

Place ingredients in a blender in the order listed. Blend until desired consistency is reached, adding water to thin out if necessary.

---

### MODIFIED VERSION
For men or those 170 pounds (77 kg) and up, increase ingredients by one-third.

---

### Nutritional Information (per serving)

Calories 309  •  Carbs 49 grams  •  Protein 17 grams  •  Fat 8 grams  •  Fiber 9 grams

# Peanut Butter and Grape Smoothie

This one makes me feel like a kid—I always used to smile when I would open my lunch box and find a PB and J sandwich. Now I can still enjoy the taste. **SERVES 1**

½ cup (125 mL) unsweetened almond milk

½ small frozen banana, chopped

½ cup (125 mL) green or red seedless grapes

1 cup (250 mL) chopped cored unpeeled apple

1 serving unsweetened protein powder

1 tablespoon (15 mL) powdered peanut butter
   (or 1½ teaspoons/7 mL reduced-fat peanut butter, or 5 peanuts)

1 tablespoon (15 mL) ground flaxseed

Ice cubes (optional)

Place ingredients in a blender in the order listed. Add ice if preferred. Blend until desired consistency is reached, adding water to thin out if necessary.

---

**MODIFIED VERSION**

For men or those 170 pounds (77 kg) and up, increase ingredients by one-third.

---

**Nutritional Information (per serving)**

Calories 324 • Carbs 45 grams • Protein 28 grams • Fat 6 grams • Fiber 8 grams

# SCRAMBLES

# Chilaquiles

Living in Los Angeles, I've fallen in love with Mexican food. With its authentic Mexican flavors, this dish tastes as good as it looks. Originally created to use up leftovers like tortillas, cheese, and shredded chicken, chilaquiles are kind of like nachos for breakfast. **SERVES 2**

Cooking oil spray

¼ cup (60 mL) chopped onion

1 cup (250 mL) chopped zucchini

1 cup (250 mL) chopped tomato

10 cups (2.4 L) fresh spinach
   (1 pound/450 g), chopped

Salt and pepper

15 baked or low-fat tortilla chips (approx.)

¼ cup (60 mL) canned black beans, drained
   and rinsed

1½ cups (375 mL) egg whites
   (12 egg whites), whisked

2 tablespoons (30 mL) shredded low-fat
   Cheddar cheese

¼ cup (60 mL) salsa

½ medium avocado, peeled and diced

Chopped fresh cilantro and hot sauce,
   for garnish

1. Preheat oven to 450°F (230°C).
2. Heat a medium nonstick ovenproof sauté pan over medium-high heat. Spray with cooking oil.
3. Add onions, zucchini, tomatoes, and spinach; sauté until vegetables are soft and spinach is wilted, about 6 minutes. Season with salt and pepper.
4. Stir in tortilla chips and black beans. Stir in egg whites. Cook, stirring often, until eggs are mostly cooked, about 4 minutes.
5. Sprinkle with cheese. Transfer pan to oven and bake until eggs are set, cheese is melted, and chips are slightly browned, 5 to 10 minutes.
6. Divide between 2 plates. Top with salsa and avocado. Garnish with cilantro and hot sauce, if desired.

**Nutritional Information (per serving)**

Calories 331 • Carbs 36 grams • Protein 32 grams • Fat 9 grams • Fiber 12 grams

# Spanish Chicken Sausage Scramble

The jalapeño in this dish gives it a bit of a kick and is also a metabolism-boosting food.   **SERVES 2**

Cooking oil spray

½ cup (125 mL) chopped onion

½ medium jalapeño pepper, seeded and finely diced

⅓ cup (75 mL) diced red bell pepper

1 cup (250 mL) finely chopped peeled sweet potato

2 ounces (55 g) chicken sausage, chopped

½ cup (125 mL) chopped tomato

½ cup (125 mL) canned chickpeas, drained and rinsed

5 cups (1.25 L) fresh spinach (12 ounces/340 g), chopped

Salt and pepper

1 cup (250 mL) egg whites (8 egg whites), whisked

2 tablespoons (30 mL) shredded low-fat Cheddar cheese

1. Heat a large nonstick sauté pan over medium-high heat. Spray with cooking oil.
2. Add onions, jalapeño, bell pepper, and sweet potatoes; sauté until vegetables are soft, about 6 minutes.
3. Add sausage; sauté until it begins to brown.
4. Stir in tomatoes, chickpeas, and spinach. Cook until spinach is wilted. Season with salt and pepper.
5. Stir in egg whites; cook, stirring constantly, until desired doneness is reached.
6. Divide between 2 plates and sprinkle with cheese.

---

**Nutritional Information (per serving)**

Calories 343  •  Carbs 48 grams  •  Protein 26 grams  •  Fat 6 grams  •  Fiber 9 grams

# Garden Vegetable Tofu Scramble

This scramble is a great way to load vegetables into your diet without having it feel like a chore. The basil adds a nice dimension to the dish. **SERVES 2**

6 ounces (170 g) extra-firm tofu

Cooking oil spray

8 medium asparagus spears, woody ends discarded, cut in 1-inch (2.5 cm) pieces

1 cup (250 mL) diced zucchini

¼ cup (60 mL) chopped green onions

½ teaspoon (2 mL) chili powder

½ cup (125 mL) chopped tomato

5 cups (1.25 L) fresh spinach (12 ounces/340 g), chopped

¼ cup (60 mL) chopped fresh basil

Salt and pepper

2 slices high-fiber bread, toasted

1. Place tofu on a plate lined with several layers of paper towels (to absorb liquid). Using a fork or potato masher, mash tofu.
2. Heat a small nonstick sauté pan over medium-high heat. Spray with cooking oil.
3. Add asparagus, zucchini, and green onions; sauté until vegetables are soft, about 5 minutes.
4. Stir in chili powder. Add tomatoes and spinach; cook, stirring occasionally, until spinach is wilted.
5. Add basil and tofu. Gently stir until heated through.
6. Season with salt and pepper. Serve with toast.

### Nutritional Information (per serving)

Calories 275 • Carbs 35 grams • Protein 24 grams • Fat 8 grams • Fiber 13 grams

# Roasted Tomato and Mushroom Scramble

This Italian-inspired scramble is especially delicious if you use fresh-cut herbs.   **SERVES 2**

4 cups (1 L) sliced mushrooms (button or shiitake)

2 cups (500 mL) halved or quartered cherry tomatoes

3 cloves garlic, crushed

3 sprigs fresh thyme

1 tablespoon (15 mL) extra-virgin olive oil

Salt and pepper

Cooking oil spray

¾ cup (175 mL) egg whites (6 egg whites)

¼ cup (60 mL) skim milk

½ cup (125 mL) shredded low-fat Cheddar cheese

1 tablespoon (15 mL) chopped fresh chives

2 slices high-fiber bread, toasted

2 tablespoons (30 mL) sugar-free fruit jam or preserves

1. Preheat oven to 400°F (200°C).
2. In a large bowl, toss mushrooms, tomatoes, garlic, and thyme sprigs with oil until evenly coated. Spread in an even layer on a baking sheet. Season with salt and pepper.
3. Roast for 12 to 15 minutes, until vegetables begin to wilt and brown.
4. Remove from oven. Discard thyme sprigs.
5. Heat a medium nonstick sauté pan over medium-high heat. Spray with cooking oil.
6. Whisk together egg whites and milk. Season with salt and pepper. Pour egg mixture into pan and cook, stirring, until completely cooked.
7. Gently fold in roasted mushroom mixture and cheese.
8. Transfer to plates and sprinkle with chopped chives. Serve with toast and jam.

### Nutritional Information (per serving)

Calories 292  •  Carbs 34 grams  •  Protein 30 grams  •  Fat 8 grams  •  Fiber 9 grams

# Smoked Salmon, Asparagus, and Goat Cheese Scramble

I love making this for guests because it tastes and looks gourmet, but it requires only a few minutes and a handful of ingredients.  **SERVES 2**

Cooking oil spray

2 tablespoons (30 mL) chopped onion

12 medium asparagus spears, woody ends discarded, very thinly sliced

5 cups (1.25 L) fresh spinach (12 ounces/340 g), chopped

3 tablespoons (45 mL) water

1 cup (250 mL) egg whites (8 egg whites)

¼ cup (60 mL) skim milk

Salt and pepper

2 tablespoons (30 mL) crumbled soft goat cheese

1 cup (250 mL) halved cherry tomatoes

3 ounces (85 g) thinly sliced smoked salmon

2 high-fiber English muffins

Chopped fresh chives, for garnish

1. Heat a large nonstick sauté pan over medium-high heat. Spray with cooking oil.
2. Add onions and asparagus; cook, stirring often, until they begin to soften, about 5 minutes.
3. Stir in spinach and water. Cover pan and cook for another 4 minutes, until asparagus is cooked through, spinach is wilted, and water has evaporated.
4. Meanwhile, whisk together egg whites and milk. Season with salt and pepper.
5. Add egg mixture to pan and gently cook, stirring constantly, until eggs are completely cooked.
6. Gently fold in goat cheese, tomatoes, and salmon.
7. Top each half of English muffins with scramble. Garnish with chopped chives, if desired.

**Nutritional Information (per serving)**

Calories 358 • Carbs 39 grams • Protein 36 grams • Fat 9 grams • Fiber 9 grams

# Green Veggie and Potato Scramble

This hearty scramble is both delicious and filling, while sneaking a variety of nutritious vegetables into your diet. It's especially good for a late Sunday breakfast with some piping-hot coffee.   **SERVES 2**

2 teaspoons (10 mL) extra-virgin olive oil

1 cup (250 mL) chopped onion

1 cup (250 mL) diced small purple or red potatoes

1 medium zucchini, chopped

2 cups (500 mL) chopped asparagus

5 cups (1.25 L) fresh spinach (12 ounces/340 g), chopped

1 cup (250 mL) egg whites (8 egg whites), whisked

Salt and pepper

1/4 cup (60 mL) shredded low-fat Cheddar cheese

2 large green onions (green and white parts), chopped

1. Heat a large nonstick sauté pan over medium-high heat. Add olive oil.
2. Add onions and potatoes; cook, stirring often, for 3 minutes.
3. Add zucchini and asparagus; cook, tossing, until they begin to caramelize, about 4 minutes.
4. Add spinach; cook, tossing, until spinach begins to wilt.
5. Stir in egg whites. Season with salt and pepper. Cook, stirring constantly, until eggs are completely cooked.
6. Divide between 2 plates and sprinkle with cheese and green onions.

**Nutritional Information (per serving)**

Calories 281  •  Carbs 33 grams  •  Protein 25 grams  •  Fat 8 grams  •  Fiber 10 grams

# Sautéed Garden
# Veggie Scramble

Another delicious scramble loaded with veggies while still tasting like comfort food. Leeks are a cousin of garlic and onion but they have a much milder flavor. **SERVES 2**

1 teaspoon (5 mL) extra-virgin olive oil

1 cup (250 mL) chopped leeks (white and pale green parts)

16 cups (3.8 L) fresh spinach (17 ounces/475 g)

Cooking oil spray

1½ cups (375 mL) chopped zucchini

2 cups (500 mL) chopped asparagus

1 cup (250 mL) chopped red bell pepper

Salt and pepper

1 cup (250 mL) egg whites (8 egg whites), whisked

2 tablespoons (30 mL) crumbled soft goat cheese

1. Heat a large nonstick sauté pan over medium-high heat. Add olive oil.
2. Add leeks and spinach; cook, stirring often, until spinach is wilted, about 5 minutes.
3. Transfer spinach mixture to a cutting board and coarsely chop.
4. Return pan to heat. Spray with cooking oil.
5. Add zucchini, asparagus, and bell pepper. Season with salt and pepper. Cook, stirring often, until beginning to brown, about 4 minutes.
6. Stir in chopped spinach mixture. Stir in egg whites. Season with salt and pepper. Cook, stirring constantly, until eggs are completely cooked.
7. Divide between 2 plates and top with goat cheese.

| Nutritional Information (per serving) |
|---|
| Calories 279 • Carbs 32 grams • Protein 29 grams • Fat 7 grams • Fiber 12 grams |

# Open-Faced Veggie Scramble Sandwich

The chickpeas (aka garbanzo beans) in this scramble make it a surprisingly hearty meal. **SERVES 2**

Cooking oil spray

¼ cup (60 mL) chopped red onion

¼ cup (60 mL) chopped bell pepper (any color)

¼ cup (60 mL) chopped zucchini

¼ cup (60 mL) canned chickpeas, drained and rinsed

1 tablespoon (15 mL) chopped fresh parsley

1 cup (250 mL) egg whites (8 egg whites), whisked

Salt and pepper

¼ cup (60 mL) shredded low-fat Cheddar cheese

¼ cup (60 mL) chopped tomato

2 slices high-fiber bread, toasted

1. Heat a large nonstick sauté pan over medium-high heat. Spray with cooking oil.
2. Add onions and bell pepper; cook, stirring often, until beginning to soften, about 4 minutes.
3. Add zucchini, chickpeas, and parsley; continue to cook for another 4 minutes.
4. Stir in egg whites. Season with salt and pepper. Cook, stirring constantly, until eggs are almost cooked.
5. Gently fold in cheese and tomatoes. Continue cooking until eggs are completely cooked.
6. Top toast with egg scramble.

**Nutritional Information (per serving)**

Calories 263 • Carbs 36 grams • Protein 28 grams • Fat 4 grams • Fiber 11 grams

# California Egg White English Muffin

Here's the perfect breakfast when you wake up hungry. A classic go-to dish that is delicious and satisfying.
**SERVES 1**

Cooking oil spray

1 whole-grain or high-fiber English muffin

6 cups (1.5 L) fresh spinach (14 ounces/400 g)

Salt and pepper

½ cup (125 mL) egg whites (4 egg whites), whisked

1 slice medium tomato

1 slice low-fat Cheddar or similar cheese

¼ medium avocado, peeled and sliced

1. Heat a small nonstick sauté pan over medium-high heat. Spray with cooking oil.
2. Meanwhile, toast English muffin.
3. Add spinach to pan; season with salt and pepper. Cook, stirring occasionally, until wilted. Remove spinach to a plate.
4. Wipe pan with paper towel, return to heat, and spray with cooking oil. Pour in egg whites. Cook, without stirring, until the bottom starts to set. Season with salt and pepper.
5. Gently lift the edges with a spatula and allow uncooked egg to flow under the cooked egg. Cook until the eggs are completely cooked through. Fold in half, then fold again into quarters.
6. Place cooked egg on one half of English muffin. Top with tomato, then hot spinach, then cheese, avocado, and finally with other half of English muffin.

---

**Nutritional Information (per serving)**

Calories 311 • Carbs 39 grams • Protein 28 grams • Fat 8 grams • Fiber 10 grams

# Italian Breakfast Frittata

*Frittata* is the Italian word for an omelet. The combo of tomato, basil, and mozzarella will whisk you away to Italy! **SERVES 2**

1 cup (250 mL) egg whites (8 egg whites)

2 tablespoons (30 mL) fat-free or low-fat cream cheese

1 tablespoon (15 mL) grated reduced-fat Parmesan cheese

1 tablespoon (15 mL) chopped fresh oregano (or 1 teaspoon/5 mL dried)

Salt and pepper

Cooking oil spray

1 cup (250 mL) chopped onion

10 cups (2.4 L) fresh spinach (1 pound/450 g), chopped

1 cup (250 mL) chopped tomato

¼ cup (60 mL) shredded fat-free mozzarella cheese

2 tablespoons (30 mL) chopped fresh basil

2 slices high-fiber bread, toasted

1. Whisk together egg whites, cream cheese, Parmesan, oregano, and salt and pepper. Set aside.
2. Heat a large nonstick sauté pan over medium-high heat. Spray with cooking oil.
3. Add onions and spinach. Season with salt and pepper. Cook, stirring occasionally, for 3 minutes.
4. Reduce heat to medium. Stir in tomatoes, then stir in egg mixture. Cook, without stirring, until the bottom is set, about 2 minutes.
5. Cover and cook until eggs are completely set, about 8 minutes. Sprinkle with mozzarella, cover, and cook for 2 more minutes.
6. Slide frittata onto a cutting board and cut into 4 wedges. Serve 2 wedges per serving, sprinkled with basil, with 1 slice of toast.

**Nutritional Information (per serving)**

Calories 306 • Carbs 39 grams • Protein 30 grams • Fat 7 grams • Fiber 11 grams

# Chicken and Egg Hash

I love this Tex-Mex scramble with a fiery hot sauce.   **SERVES 2**

2 teaspoons (10 mL) olive oil

1 cup (250 mL) chopped onion

1 cup (250 mL) diced peeled sweet potato

1 cup (250 mL) diced red bell pepper

1 cup (250 mL) diced green bell pepper

1 cup (250 mL) canned pinto beans, drained and rinsed

3 ounces (85 g) cooked skinless chicken breast, chopped

Salt and pepper

½ cup (125 mL) egg whites (4 egg whites), whisked

Hot sauce and chopped fresh cilantro, for garnish

1. Heat a medium nonstick sauté pan over medium-high heat. Add olive oil.
2. Add onions and sweet potatoes; sauté until onions and potatoes begin to brown, about 4 minutes.
3. Stir in red and green bell peppers. Sauté until potatoes are beginning to become tender.
4. Stir in beans and chicken. Season with salt and pepper.
5. Stir in egg whites. Cook, stirring, until eggs are completely cooked through, 2 to 4 minutes.
6. Divide eggs between 2 plates and garnish with hot sauce and cilantro, if desired.

**Nutritional Information (per serving)**

Calories 361  •  Carbs 48 grams  •  Protein 28 grams  •  Fat 8 grams  •  Fiber 12 grams

# Easy Rancheros

Black beans have been a longtime staple in Mexican and Central and South American cuisines, and with good reason—they're filling and nutritious. Easy rancheros is often smothered in sauce and grease, but this much healthier version still hits the spot.  **SERVES 2**

Cooking oil spray

2 large eggs

Salt and pepper

1 cup (250 mL) canned black beans, drained and rinsed

½ cup (125 mL) any shredded low-fat cheese or blend

¼ cup (60 mL) fat-free salsa

Chopped jalapeño pepper and fresh cilantro, for garnish

2 low-carb high-fiber tortillas, warmed

1. Heat a medium nonstick sauté pan over medium-high heat. Spray with cooking oil.
2. Whisk eggs and season with salt and pepper. Add to pan and cook, stirring constantly.
3. When eggs are three-quarters cooked, stir in beans and cheese. Continue to cook, stirring, until eggs are completely cooked.
4. Fold in salsa, if desired, or serve on the side.
5. Divide eggs between 2 plates. Garnish with chopped jalapeño and cilantro, if desired. Serve with warm tortillas.

**Nutritional Information (per serving)**

Calories 295  •  Carbs 33 grams  •  Protein 26 grams  •  Fat 10 grams  •  Fiber 15 grams

# Green Eggs and Ham

Kids and adults alike will eat spinach with no complaint when it's disguised in this Dr. Seuss treat.
**SERVES 2**

5 cups (1.25 L) fresh spinach (12 ounces/340 g), chopped

¾ cup (175 mL) egg whites (6 egg whites), whisked

Salt and pepper

Cooking oil spray

3 ounces (85 g) extra-lean deli ham, sliced or chopped

¼ cup (60 mL) shredded part-skim mozzarella cheese

2 slices high-fiber bread

2 tablespoons (30 mL) sugar-free fruit jam

2 medium plum tomatoes, sliced or quartered

1. In a blender, combine spinach and egg whites. Blend until mixture is a smooth green liquid. Season with salt and pepper.
2. Heat a small nonstick sauté pan over medium heat. Spray with cooking oil.
3. Pour spinach mixture into pan and cook, stirring constantly, until eggs are almost cooked and excess water from spinach has evaporated, about 10 minutes.
4. Just before eggs are cooked, fold in ham and cheese. Continue to cook, stirring, until eggs are completely cooked through.
5. Meanwhile, toast bread and spread with jam.
6. Divide eggs between 2 plates. Sprinkle a pinch of salt over tomatoes and serve on the side with the toast.

**Nutritional Information (per serving)**

Calories 333 • Carbs 36 grams • Protein 33 grams • Fat 9 grams • Fiber 8 grams

# Spanish Breakfast Stew

This dish is as good to look at as it is to eat. And you'll earn major points with your partner by making this for breakfast in bed.  **SERVES 2**

1 teaspoon (5 mL) cumin seeds
   (or ground cumin, but do not toast)

1 teaspoon (5 mL) extra-virgin olive oil

1 cup (250 mL) chopped onion

1 clove garlic, minced

1 cup (250 mL) halved cherry tomatoes

8 cups (2 L) fresh spinach (roughly
   1 pound/450 g), chopped

1 tablespoon (15 mL) paprika
   (preferably smoked)

1 cup (250 mL) canned chickpeas, drained
   and rinsed

2 cups (500 mL) fat-free vegetable or
   chicken broth

Salt and pepper

Cooking oil spray

2 large eggs

1 slice high-fiber bread, grilled or toasted,
   cut in half diagonally

1. Heat a large nonstick sauté pan over medium-high heat. Add cumin seeds (if using) and toast, stirring, until fragrant, about 1 minute.
2. Add olive oil. When hot, add onions and garlic; sauté until starting to brown, about 4 minutes.
3. Add tomatoes; sauté until blistering, about 3 minutes.
4. Add spinach; cook, stirring often, until wilted.
5. Stir in ground cumin (if using), paprika, chickpeas, and broth. Cover, reduce heat to low, and cook for 10 minutes, stirring occasionally. Season with salt and pepper.
6. Heat a small nonstick sauté pan over medium-high heat. Spray with cooking oil.
7. Fry eggs until desired doneness, about 2 minutes for over easy. Season with salt and pepper.
8. Divide stew between 2 bowls and top each serving with a fried egg. Serve toast on the side for dipping.

**Nutritional Information (per serving)**

Calories 358  •  Carbs 52 grams  •  Protein 21 grams  •  Fat 10 grams  •  Fiber 14 grams

# Egg in a Hole
# with Grapefruit

This classic American breakfast is hearty but light—good for before a hike or a day of traveling.   **SERVES 2**

2 slices high-fiber bread

1 teaspoon (5 mL) extra-virgin olive oil

4 large egg whites

Salt and pepper

2 slices fat-free cheese singles

1 medium grapefruit, halved crosswise

1. Using a cookie cutter or drinking glass, cut a hole from the middle of each slice of bread. Set aside bread circles.
2. Heat a large nonstick sauté pan over medium heat. Add olive oil.
3. Arrange bread slices and circles in pan, then turn so both sides of bread are oiled.
4. Slide 2 egg whites into each hole. Season with salt and pepper. Cook until bread is golden brown on the bottom, about 2 minutes. Turn bread and circles. Top bread slices with cheese, cover, and continue to cook for 2 minutes. Serve with grapefruit and bread circles.

**Nutritional Information (per serving)**

Calories 332  •  Carbs 52 grams  •  Protein 27 grams  •  Fat 7 grams  •  Fiber 10 grams

# SALADS

# BBQ Farro Salad

Farro is a power grain with ancient roots. It tastes earthy and nutty and delicious. In this salad, it soaks up the tangy flavors of the barbecue dressing while providing protein, fiber, magnesium, and vitamins A, B, C, and E. **SERVES 2**

10 cups (2.4 L) fresh spinach (1 pound/450 g), chopped

1½ cups (375 mL) cooked farro

1 cup (250 mL) fresh corn kernels

1 cup (250 mL) shelled edamame, cooked

1 cup (250 mL) halved cherry tomatoes

¼ cup (60 mL) chopped red onion

1 tablespoon (15 mL) cider vinegar or red wine vinegar

1 tablespoon (15 mL) fat-free ranch dressing

1 tablespoon (15 mL) barbecue sauce

Salt and pepper

1. In a large bowl, combine spinach, farro, corn, edamame, tomatoes, onions, vinegar, ranch dressing, and barbecue sauce; toss to coat. Season with salt and pepper.
2. Refrigerate for at least 30 minutes before serving.

**Nutritional Information (per serving)**

Calories 373 • Carbs 64 grams • Protein 22 grams • Fat 7 grams • Fiber 9 grams

# Baked Tofu Summer Salad

I love taking this salad to barbecues. It's always a huge hit. The natural sweetness of the corn adds a burst of flavor, while the jalapeño provides a hint of spiciness, making this an exciting and delicious dish. **SERVES 2**

18 fresh green beans, trimmed and cut in 1-inch (2.5 cm) pieces

½ cup (125 mL) fresh corn kernels

½ cup (125 mL) halved cherry tomatoes

¼ cup (60 mL) canned or thawed frozen lima beans

¼ cup (60 mL) diced avocado

¼ cup (60 mL) finely chopped red onion

¼ medium jalapeño pepper, seeded and finely diced

8 ounces (225 g) extra-firm tofu

Cooking oil spray

**DRESSING**

1 tablespoon (15 mL) red wine vinegar

1 tablespoon (15 mL) canola or other vegetable oil

1 tablespoon (15 mL) chopped or thinly sliced fresh basil

½ teaspoon (2 mL) stevia or sweetener of your choice

Salt and pepper

1. For the dressing: In a large bowl, combine vinegar, oil, basil, and stevia; whisk until blended. Season with salt and pepper.
2. Add green beans, corn, tomatoes, lima beans, avocado, onions, and jalapeño. Toss with dressing. Let marinate at room temperature for at least 1 hour.
3. Preheat oven to 400°F (200°C).
4. Wrap tofu in 4 or 5 layers of paper towels and press down to squeeze excess moisture from the tofu. Cut tofu into cubes.
5. Lightly spray tofu with cooking oil. Arrange in a single layer on a baking sheet. Bake, flipping halfway through, until golden brown and just crisp, about 40 minutes.
6. Toss tofu with salad and divide between 2 plates.

| Nutritional Information (per serving) |
| --- |

Calories 350 • Carbs 45 grams • Protein 24 grams • Fat 9 grams • Fiber 11 grams

# Summer Shrimp Salad

This is a refreshing and clean salad. Experiment with other fresh herbs for a totally different flavor.
**SERVES 2**

6 ounces (170 g) peeled cooked shrimp, chopped

2 cups (500 mL) cubed seeded watermelon

2 cups (500 mL) chopped unpeeled English cucumber

1 cup (250 mL) fresh corn kernels

¼ cup (60 mL) chopped red onion

½ medium avocado, peeled and diced

1 small jalapeño pepper, seeded and finely chopped

4 cups (1 L) watercress, coarse stems removed

Chopped fresh cilantro, basil, and/or mint

**DRESSING**

2 tablespoons (30 mL) cider or other vinegar

2 teaspoons (10 mL) dried cilantro

1 teaspoon (5 mL) canola oil

½ teaspoon (2 mL) stevia or sweetener of your choice

Juice of 1 lime

Salt and pepper

1. For the dressing: In a small bowl, combine vinegar, cilantro, oil, stevia, and lime juice; whisk until blended. Season with salt and pepper.
2. In a medium bowl, combine shrimp, watermelon, cucumber, corn, onions, avocado, and jalapeño.
3. Add dressing and toss to coat. Season with salt and pepper.
4. Divide watercress between 2 plates. Spoon salad mixture over watercress. Sprinkle salad with fresh herbs.

**Nutritional Information (per serving)**

Calories 355 • Carbs 52 grams • Protein 28 grams • Fat 8 grams • Fiber 10 grams

# Salmon and Kale Salad

Kale deserves its popularity—it's loaded with fiber and nutrients and is always in season.   **SERVES 2**

½ teaspoon (2 mL) paprika

½ teaspoon (2 mL) cayenne

Salt and pepper

2 skinless salmon fillets (2 ounces/55 g each)

Cooking oil spray

6 cups (1.5 L) shredded kale

1 cup (250 mL) roasted cubed butternut squash

⅔ cup (150 mL) cooked pearl barley

**DRESSING**

2 tablespoons (30 mL) sherry vinegar or red wine vinegar

2 teaspoons (10 mL) walnut oil or vegetable oil

1 teaspoon (5 mL) stevia or sweetener of your choice

Salt and pepper

1. For the dressing: In a large bowl, combine vinegar, oil, and stevia; whisk until blended. Season with salt and pepper. Set aside.
2. Stir together paprika, cayenne, and salt and pepper to taste. Sprinkle over both sides of salmon.
3. Heat a medium nonstick sauté pan over medium-high heat. Spray with cooking oil.
4. Sear salmon on both sides, turning once, until middle is cooked through, 4 to 5 minutes per side.
5. Add kale, squash, and barley to dressing; toss well. Season with a pinch of salt.
6. Divide salad between 2 plates and top with salmon.

**Nutritional Information (per serving)**

Calories 344 • Carbs 48 grams • Protein 21 grams • Fat 10 grams • Fiber 13 grams

# Salmon, Kale, and Roasted Sweet Potato Salad with Miso Vinaigrette

The crunchy texture of kale goes perfectly with the sweet starchiness of sweet potatoes in this Asian-inspired recipe. **SERVES 2**

Cooking oil spray

2 tablespoons (30 mL) white miso paste

1 tablespoon (15 mL) low-sodium soy sauce

1 tablespoon (15 mL) water

1 teaspoon (5 mL) sesame oil

Salt and pepper

2 cups (500 mL) peeled sweet potato cut in half-moons ¼ inch (5 mm) thick (about 3 medium)

2 skinless salmon fillets (2 ounces/55 g each) or 4 ounces (115 g) grilled skinless chicken breast, chopped

6 cups (1.5 L) shredded kale

1. Preheat oven to 400°F (200°C). Spray a baking sheet with cooking oil.
2. In a small bowl, stir together miso, soy sauce, water, and sesame oil until smooth. Season vinaigrette with salt and pepper.
3. In a large bowl, toss sweet potatoes with half of the vinaigrette, then arrange in a single layer on the baking sheet. Set aside the bowl. Season potatoes with salt and pepper. Roast, turning once halfway through, until brown, about 15 minutes. Let cool for 15 minutes.
4. Meanwhile, season both sides of salmon with salt and pepper.
5. Heat a medium nonstick sauté pan over medium-high heat. Spray with cooking oil.
6. Add salmon and cook, turning once, until cooked through, 4 to 5 minutes per side. Set salmon aside.
7. In the large bowl, toss kale with remaining vinaigrette.
8. Divide kale between 2 plates. Top with sweet potatoes and then with salmon.

| Nutritional Information (per serving) |
| --- |

Calories 375 • Carbs 56 grams • Protein 22 grams • Fat 9 grams • Fiber 12 grams

# Summer Grilled Salmon Panzanella Salad

This bread salad is a true taste of Italy. Traditionally made with anchovies, it's an Italian classic.
**SERVES 2**

2 slices whole-grain sprouted bread, cut in 1-inch (2.5 cm) cubes

2 cups (500 mL) tomatoes cut in 1-inch (2.5 cm) cubes

2 cups (500 mL) unpeeled English cucumber cut in 1-inch (2.5 cm) cubes

¼ cup (60 mL) thinly sliced red onion

5 fresh basil leaves, thinly sliced

2 skinless salmon fillets (3 ounces/85 g each)

Cooking oil spray

5 cups (1.25 L) baby arugula

**DRESSING**

4 green olives, pitted and chopped

4 teaspoons (20 mL) red wine vinegar

1½ teaspoons (7 mL) capers, rinsed and chopped

1 teaspoon (5 mL) extra-virgin olive oil

Salt and pepper

1. For the dressing: In a large bowl, combine olives, vinegar, and capers. Whisk in oil until well blended. Season with salt and pepper.
2. Add bread, tomatoes, cucumber, onions, and basil; toss well. Let sit while you grill the fish so the bread absorbs some of the juices.
3. Season both sides of salmon with salt and pepper.
4. Spray cooking oil on grill rack (or heat a medium nonstick sauté pan and spray pan). Grill salmon, turning once, until cooked through, 4 to 5 minutes per side.
5. Divide arugula between 2 plates. Top with bread salad, then top with salmon.

**Nutritional Information (per serving)**

Calories 314 • Carbs 30 grams • Protein 26 grams • Fat 11 grams • Fiber 7 grams

# Smoked Turkey Spinach Salad

This simple salad makes a perfect bag lunch to take to work or school, because it's even better after the ingredients have had a chance to marinate a little.  **SERVES 2**

3 ounces (85 g) lean smoked turkey, sliced
  or chopped

¾ cup (175 mL) shredded low-fat cheese

¾ cup (175 mL) fresh corn kernels

½ cup (125 mL) canned black beans, drained
  and rinsed

½ cup (125 mL) halved cherry tomatoes

½ cup (125 mL) chopped bell pepper
  (any color)

¼ cup (60 mL) finely chopped red onion

2 cups (500 mL) fresh baby spinach

**DRESSING**

2 tablespoons (30 mL) chopped fresh cilantro

2 tablespoons (30 mL) low-sodium canned
  or fresh tomato juice

1½ teaspoons (7 mL) minced garlic

1½ teaspoons (7 mL) extra-virgin olive oil

1½ teaspoons (7 mL) sherry vinegar or
  other vinegar

Juice of ½ lemon

Salt and pepper

1. For the dressing: In a large bowl, combine cilantro, tomato juice, garlic, olive oil, vinegar, and lemon juice; whisk until well blended. Season with salt and pepper.
2. Add turkey, cheese, corn, beans, tomatoes, bell pepper, and onions. Toss well.
3. Divide spinach between 2 plates. Top with turkey salad.

**Nutritional Information (per serving)**

**Calories 316  •  Carbs 34 grams  •  Protein 29 grams  •  Fat 8 grams  •  Fiber 9 grams**

# Nectarine Salad with Grilled Chicken and Chickpeas

The creaminess of the goat cheese and the tartness of the nectarine is a match made in heaven. Peach, pear, apple, and plum work just as well in this satisfying salad. **SERVES 2**

8 cups (2 L) fresh baby spinach (12 ounces/ 300 g)

1 cup (250 mL) canned chickpeas, drained and rinsed

1 cup (250 mL) chopped or thinly sliced nectarine

4 ounces (115 g) grilled skinless chicken breast, sliced

2 tablespoons (30 mL) crumbled soft goat cheese

**DRESSING**

2 tablespoons (30 mL) balsamic vinegar

2 teaspoons (10 mL) olive oil

Salt and pepper

1. For the dressing: In a large bowl, whisk together vinegar and oil until blended. Season with salt and pepper.
2. Add spinach and chickpeas; toss to coat.
3. Divide salad between 2 plates. Top with nectarine, then chicken, then goat cheese. Season with salt and pepper.

**Nutritional Information (per serving)**

Calories 361 • Carbs 43 grams • Protein 25 grams • Fat 11 grams • Fiber 10 grams

# Asian Chicken Salad

Many restaurants load up Asian chicken salad with unnecessary fat and sugar, often serving up a dish with more than 500 calories. Try this lighter version—you won't miss a thing!  **SERVES 2**

4 small wonton wrappers, sliced in thin strips

Cooking oil spray

Pinch of salt

4 ounces (115 g) cooked skinless chicken breast, shredded or "pulled"

4 cups (1 L) chopped or shredded romaine lettuce

3 cups (750 mL) shredded red, green, or napa cabbage

1 cup (250 mL) shredded carrots

1 cup (250 mL) diced red bell pepper

20 medium snow peas, thinly sliced

2 large green onions, thinly sliced

½ cup (125 mL) drained canned unsweetened mandarin orange segments

1 teaspoon (5 mL) each chopped fresh mint, basil, and cilantro

**DRESSING**

2 tablespoons (30 mL) rice vinegar

1 tablespoon (15 mL) low-sodium soy sauce

2 teaspoons (10 mL) minced peeled fresh ginger

2 teaspoons (10 mL) orange juice

2 teaspoons (10 mL) coconut oil or any vegetable oil

1 teaspoon (5 mL) stevia or sweetener of your choice

Salt and pepper

1. Preheat oven to 450°F (230°C).
2. Spread wonton strips on a cookie sheet and spray lightly with cooking oil. Cook, turning once halfway through, until browned and crispy, about 6 minutes. Remove from oven and sprinkle with a pinch of salt.
3. In a large bowl, combine chicken, lettuce, cabbage, carrots, bell pepper, snow peas, and green onions; toss lightly.
4. For the dressing: In a small bowl, combine rice vinegar, soy sauce, ginger, orange juice, oil, and stevia; whisk to blend. Season with salt and pepper.
5. Pour dressing over salad. Toss lightly to coat.
6. Divide salad between 2 plates. Top with mandarins, crispy wonton strips, and chopped herbs (if using).

## Nutritional Information (per serving)

Calories 324  •  Carbs 40 grams  •  Protein 25 grams  •  Fat 8 grams  •  Fiber 10 grams

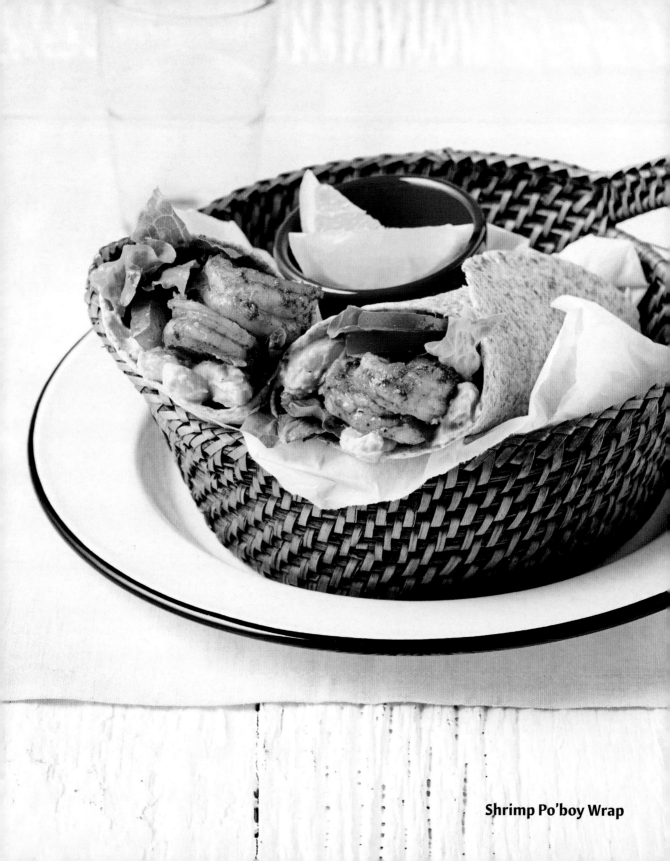

**Shrimp Po'boy Wrap**

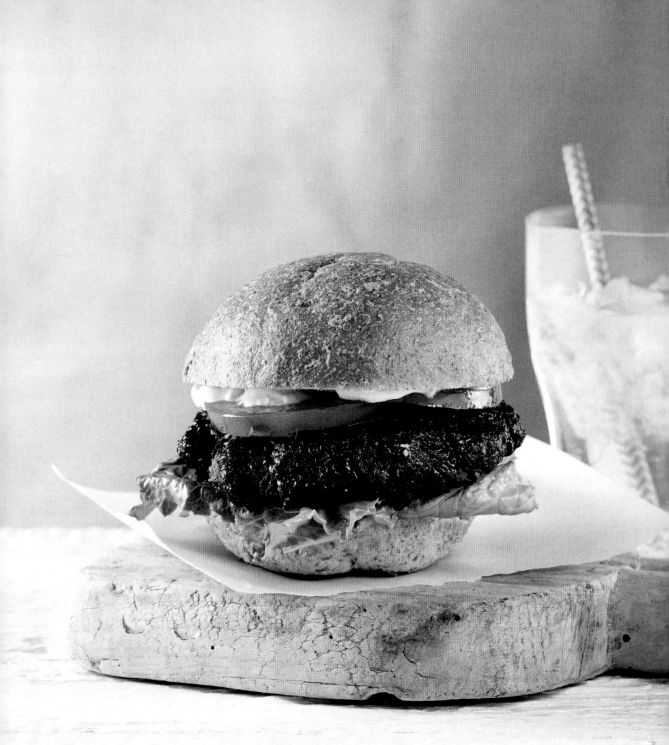

**Spicy Black Bean Beet Burger**

**Tomato and Green Olive Pizza**

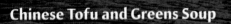

Chinese Tofu and Greens Soup

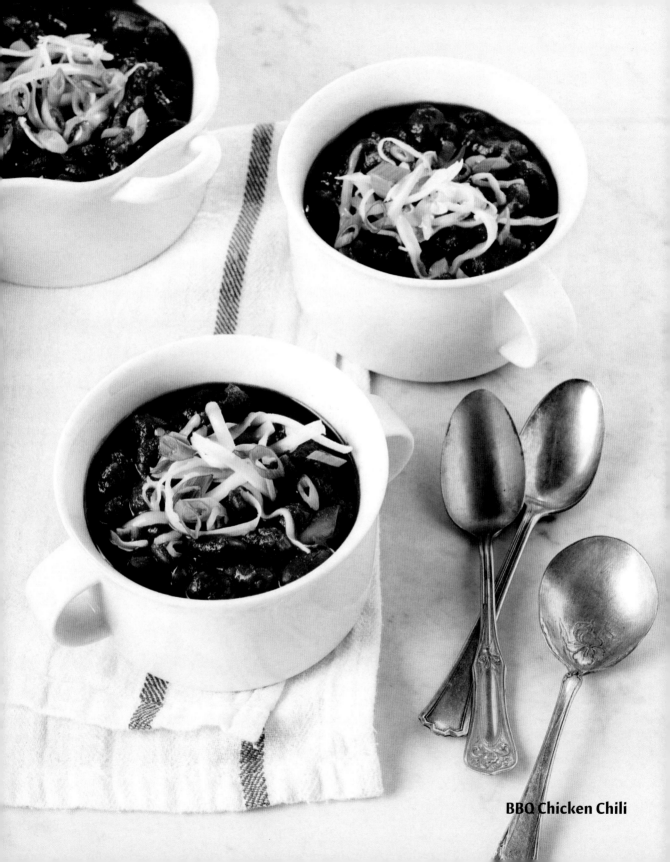

BBQ Chicken Chili

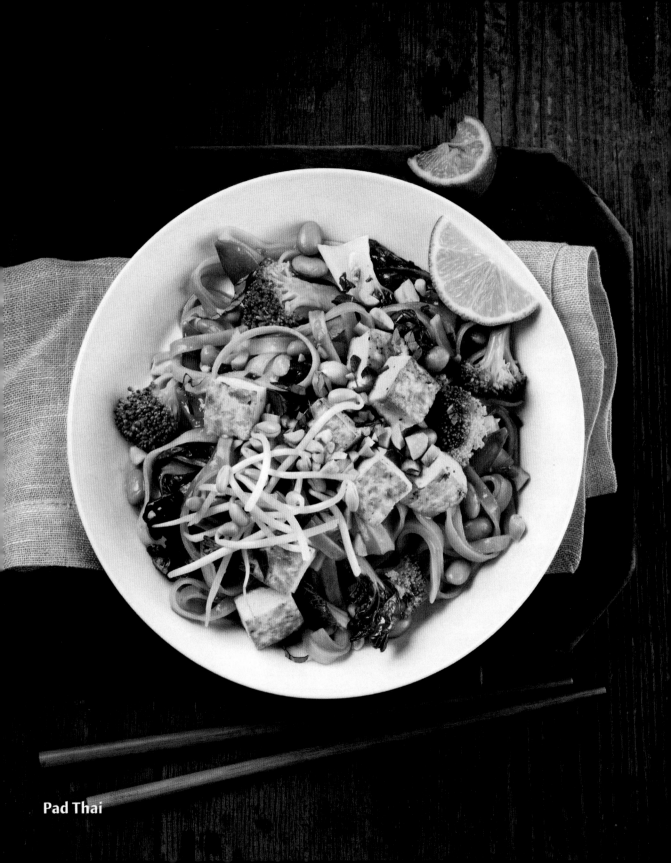

Pad Thai

Steak and Veggie Stir-Fry

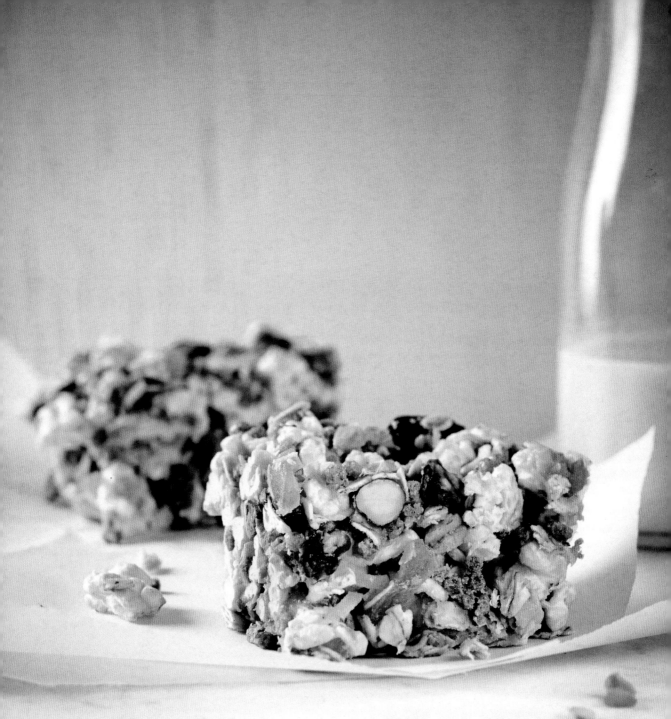

**Fruit and Nut Popcorn Bars**

# Chicken Taco Salad

Taco night is back on the menu thanks to this nutritious approach.  **SERVES 2**

Cooking oil spray

¼ cup (60 mL) chopped onion

4 ounces (115 g) ground chicken breast or
other lean protein

2 teaspoons (10 mL) taco seasoning mix

2 tablespoons (30 mL) water

1½ cups (375 mL) low-fat refried black beans

4 cups (1 L) chopped or shredded romaine
lettuce

1 cup (250 mL) chopped canned or cooked
(or shredded raw) beets

½ cup (125 mL) chopped tomato

¼ cup (60 mL) fresh corn kernels

**DRESSING**

¼ cup (60 mL) cider vinegar or other vinegar

1 teaspoon (5 mL) olive oil

½ teaspoon (2 mL) ground chipotle chili
(or 1 teaspoon/5 mL finely chopped
canned chipotle in adobo sauce)

½ teaspoon (2 mL) stevia or sweetener of
your choice

Salt and pepper

1. For the dressing: In a large bowl, whisk together vinegar, oil, chipotle, and stevia. Season with salt and pepper. Set aside.
2. Heat a medium nonstick sauté pan over medium-high heat. Spray with cooking oil.
3. Add onions and chicken; sauté until chicken is cooked through and starting to brown, about 6 minutes. Add taco seasoning and water; stir to coat. Cook, stirring often, for another 5 minutes. Transfer chicken mixture to a plate and return pan to heat.
4. Add beans to pan and cook until warmed through, about 4 minutes. Divide beans between 2 plates. Let cool slightly.
5. Add romaine, beets, and tomatoes to dressing and toss to coat well. Top beans evenly with salad.
6. Top salad with chicken, then with corn.

**Nutritional Information (per serving)**

Calories 366  •  Carbs 48 grams  •  Protein 25 grams  •  Fat 8 grams  •  Fiber 13 grams

# Hearty Grain Salad

I love the satisfying sweetness of this delicious high-fiber dish.  **SERVES 2**

4 cups (1 L) shredded kale

4 ounces (115 g) cooked skinless chicken breast, chopped or shredded

½ cup (125 mL) cooked pearl barley

½ cup (125 mL) unsweetened dried cranberries

¼ medium avocado, peeled and cubed

2 tablespoons (30 mL) sunflower seeds

**DRESSING**

1 tablespoon (15 mL) balsamic vinegar

1 teaspoon (5 mL) pure maple syrup or sweetener of your choice

Juice of 1 lemon

Salt and pepper

1. For the dressing: In a large bowl, combine vinegar, maple syrup, and lemon juice; whisk until blended. Season with salt and pepper.
2. Add kale and toss with dressing.
3. Divide between 2 plates. Top kale evenly with chicken, barley, cranberries, avocado, and sunflower seeds.

**Nutritional Information (per serving)**

Calories 317 • Carbs 41 grams • Protein 21 grams • Fat 10 grams • Fiber 12 grams

# Bean Salad
# with Grilled Chicken

I never get tired of this salad, which comes together in minutes with common pantry items. I make it whenever we have leftover chicken or turkey.  **SERVES 2**

1½ cups (375 mL) assorted canned beans (such as black, pinto, white, kidney, chickpeas), drained and rinsed

1 cup (250 mL) halved cherry tomatoes

2 tablespoons (30 mL) low-fat herbed or other low-fat vinaigrette

Salt and pepper

4 cups (1 L) shredded romaine lettuce

4 ounces (115 g) grilled skinless chicken breast, thinly sliced

1. Combine beans, tomatoes, and vinaigrette in a medium bowl. Season with salt and pepper. Toss to coat. Let sit in refrigerator for at least 20 minutes.
2. Divide romaine between 2 plates. Top with bean salad, then with chicken.

**Nutritional Information (per serving)**

Calories 312  •  Carbs 42 grams  •  Protein 26 grams  •  Fat 5 grams  •  Fiber 13 grams

# Spring Vegetable Salad with Chicken

Pumpkin seeds (or pepitas) are a rich source of iron and magnesium. I like raw pepitas in this recipe, but roasted ones will do; just watch the sodium content on the store-bought variety. **SERVES 2**

2 cups (500 mL) green beans, trimmed

2 small zucchini

6 cups (1.5 L) mixed salad greens

4 tablespoons (60 mL) low-fat vinaigrette

Salt and pepper

2 cups (500 mL) shredded carrots

2 thin slices red onion

4 ounces (115 g) grilled skinless chicken breast, thinly sliced or chopped

2 tablespoons (30 mL) crumbled soft goat cheese

2 tablespoons (30 mL) pumpkin seeds, toasted

1. Bring a large pot of salted water to a boil. Add green beans and cook until bright green and tender-crisp, about 1½ minutes. Drain beans and plunge into ice water to stop the cooking. When cool, remove from ice water (reserving the water), pat dry, and set aside.
2. Using a vegetable peeler, peel lengthwise ribbons of zucchini that are thin enough to curl or fold over without breaking. Place ribbons in ice water until ready to use.
3. In a large bowl, lightly toss salad greens with 2 tablespoons (30 mL) of the vinaigrette and a pinch of salt and pepper. Divide between 2 plates.
4. Drain zucchini and pat dry. In the same bowl, combine zucchini, green beans, carrots, onion, and remaining 2 tablespoons (30 mL) dressing. Toss well. Season with salt and pepper.
5. Top salad greens with vegetable mixture, then top with chicken, goat cheese, and pumpkin seeds.

**Nutritional Information (per serving)**

Calories 315 • Carbs 35 grams • Protein 22 grams • Fat 10 grams • Fiber 13 grams

# Apple, Quinoa, and Blue Cheese Salad

A summery alternative to the standard chicken or Waldorf salad.  **SERVES 2**

½ cup (125 mL) nonfat plain yogurt

2 tablespoons (30 mL) crumbled reduced-fat blue cheese

1 tablespoon (15 mL) chopped fresh tarragon (more for garnish, if desired)

1 tablespoon (15 mL) cider vinegar or red or white wine vinegar

Salt and pepper

1 large unpeeled apple, diced

1 cup (250 mL) diced celery

4 ounces (115 g) cooked skinless chicken breast, diced

8 cups (2 L) arugula

1½ cups (375 mL) cooked quinoa or other cooked whole grain (such as bulgur or barley)

1. In a small bowl, combine yogurt, blue cheese, tarragon, and vinegar. Season with salt and pepper. Stir together well. Chill dressing for at least 20 minutes.
2. In a large bowl, combine apple, celery, and chicken. Add dressing and toss well.
3. Divide arugula between 2 plates. Top evenly with quinoa, then with chicken salad. Garnish with tarragon, if desired.

### Nutritional Information (per serving)

Calories 385  •  Carbs 57 grams  •  Protein 26 grams  •  Fat 6 grams  •  Fiber 11 grams

# Italian Chopped Salad

My tribute to Los Angeles's most famed salad, La Scala's Chopped Salad.  **SERVES 2**

5 cups (1.25 L) finely chopped romaine lettuce

2 cups (500 mL) finely chopped fresh spinach

4 ounces (115 g) cooked skinless chicken breast, chopped

1 ounce (28 g) sliced hard Italian salami, cut in thin strips

1 medium unpeeled English cucumber, chopped (about 2 cups/500 mL)

5 fresh basil leaves, chopped

2 cups (500 mL) halved or quartered cherry tomatoes

½ cup (125 mL) canned chickpeas, drained and rinsed

2 tablespoons (30 mL) shredded part-skim mozzarella cheese

**VINAIGRETTE**

1 tablespoon (15 mL) chopped fresh basil

1 tablespoon (15 mL) grated reduced-fat Parmesan cheese

1 tablespoon (15 mL) red wine vinegar

1 teaspoon (5 mL) Dijon mustard

Juice of 1 lemon

Salt and pepper

1. For the vinaigrette: In a small bowl, combine basil, Parmesan, vinegar, mustard, and lemon juice. Whisk until well blended. Season with salt and pepper. Set aside.
2. In a large bowl, toss together romaine and spinach. Divide between 2 plates.
3. In the same bowl, combine chicken, salami, cucumber, basil, tomatoes, chickpeas, and mozzarella; toss well. Spoon mixture over salad greens. Season with salt and pepper.
4. Dress salad with vinaigrette right before serving.

---

**Nutritional Information (per serving)**

Calories 320  •  Carbs 35 grams  •  Protein 28 grams  •  Fat 10 grams  •  Fiber 9 grams

# SANDWICHES, WRAPS, AND BURGERS

# California Grilled Cheese

Comfort food need not be forbidden. Here it is at its finest—warm grilled cheese has never been so tasty and healthy.  **SERVES 1**

2 slices high-fiber bread

3 slices low-fat Cheddar and/or Colby cheese

1/8 medium avocado, peeled and thinly sliced

4 slices medium tomato

Cooking oil spray

1. On 1 slice of bread, layer 1 slice of cheese, avocado, second slice of cheese, tomato, and last slice of cheese. Top with second slice of bread.
2. Heat a small nonstick sauté pan over medium heat. Spray with cooking oil. Spray both sides of sandwich.
3. Place sandwich in pan and cover with lid. Heat each side until bread is toasted and cheese is melted. Lower temperature if bread is browning too quickly.

| Nutritional Information (per serving) |
| --- |

Calories 294 • Carbs 32 grams • Protein 27 grams • Fat 10 grams • Fiber 12 grams

# BLAST Sandwich

Instead of a tired old BLT, try my BLAST (Bacon, Lettuce, Avocado, Sprouts, and Tomato). Look for hummus with 2 grams of protein per 30 calories. **SERVES 1**

¼ cup (60 mL) fat-free hummus

2 slices high-fiber bread, toasted

1 large romaine lettuce leaf

2 slices medium tomato

½ cup (125 mL) alfalfa sprouts

2 slices cooked turkey bacon

¼ medium avocado, peeled and sliced

1. Spread half the hummus on each slice of toast.
2. On 1 slice of toast, layer lettuce, tomato, sprouts, turkey bacon, and avocado. Top with second slice of toast.

**Nutritional Information (per serving)**

Calories 299 • Carbs 41 grams • Protein 24 grams • Fat 9 grams • Fiber 18 grams

# Roast Turkey, Brie, and Apple Sandwich

The delicious combination of turkey, Brie cheese, and apple makes this sandwich one of my favorites. For variety, try different types of high-fiber bread and apples. **SERVES 2**

4 slices high-fiber bread, toasted

6 ounces (170 g) thinly sliced roasted turkey breast

2 slices (½ inch/1 cm wide each) Brie cheese (2 ounces/55 g)

1 small unpeeled apple, cored and sliced

2 cups (500 mL) baby arugula

Salt and pepper

4 teaspoons (20 mL) honey mustard

1. Top 2 slices of toast with turkey, cheese, apple, and arugula. Season with salt and pepper.
2. Spread mustard on the other 2 slices of toast and place over filling.

### Nutritional Information (per serving)

Calories 330 • Carbs 43 grams • Protein 26 grams • Fat 10 grams • Fiber 12 grams

# Spicy Tempeh Wrap

Tempeh, like its cousin tofu, is a soy product, but it's firmer and more chewy (like meat). It's also higher in protein and fiber than most tofu.   **SERVES 2**

Cooking oil spray

6 ounces (170 g) tempeh, chopped

¼ cup (60 mL) canned enchilada sauce or Mexican spicy marinade

2 low-carb high-fiber tortillas

2 cups (500 mL) shredded romaine lettuce

1 cup (250 mL) chopped tomato

1. Heat a medium nonstick sauté pan over medium-high heat. Spray with cooking oil.
2. Add tempeh; sauté until tempeh begins to brown and crisp.
3. Add enchilada sauce; cook, stirring often, until tempeh is completely glazed in sauce. Remove from heat.
4. Warm tortillas (heat in a sauté pan over medium heat until pliable, or microwave for 30 seconds).
5. Top tortillas with lettuce, tomatoes, and cooked tempeh. Fold or roll up.

**Nutritional Information (per serving)**

Calories 292  •  Carbs 40 grams  •  Protein 26 grams  •  Fat 10 grams  •  Fiber 22 grams

# Spicy Hummus Wrap

This wrap is packed with super-foods. Even better, recent research shows that eating avocado with a meal helps you absorb the nutrients more easily.  **SERVES 2**

1 cup (250 mL) fat-free hummus

1 cup (250 mL) drained canned artichoke hearts

Sriracha sauce

2 low-carb high-fiber tortillas

2 cups (500 mL) baby arugula

1 cup (250 mL) grated carrots

¼ medium avocado, peeled and sliced

Salt and pepper

1. In a food processor, combine hummus, artichokes, and Sriracha sauce to taste. Process until smooth.
2. Warm tortillas (heat in a sauté pan over medium heat until pliable, or microwave for 30 seconds).
3. Spread hummus mixture over tortillas. Top with arugula, carrots, and avocado. Season with salt and pepper. Fold or roll up.

**Nutritional Information (per serving)**

Calories 304  •  Carbs 53 grams  •  Protein 21 grams  •  Fat 7 grams  •  Fiber 16 grams

# BBQ Chicken Wrap

I use cabbage instead of lettuce in this wrap to add some extra crunch.  **SERVES** 1

2 ounces (55 g) cooked skinless chicken breast, chopped

2 tablespoons (30 mL) barbecue sauce

1 low-carb high-fiber tortilla

½ cup (125 mL) shredded cabbage (any kind)

¼ cup (60 mL) fresh corn kernels

½ cup (125 mL) diced tomato

2 tablespoons (30 mL) crumbled reduced-fat feta cheese

1. Heat a small nonstick sauté pan over medium heat. Add chicken and barbecue sauce. Cook, stirring occasionally, until heated through.
2. Warm tortilla (heat in a sauté pan over medium heat until pliable, or microwave for 30 seconds).
3. Top tortilla with chicken, cabbage, corn, tomatoes, and feta. Fold or roll up.

**Nutritional Information (per serving)**

Calories 284  •  **Carbs 36 grams**  •  **Protein 29 grams**  •  **Fat 9 grams**  •  **Fiber 15 grams**

# Miso Chicken Salad Wrap

This miso wrap is a go-to for my clients when they crave Chinese food. If you are using reduced-fat mayonnaise, make sure it's canola oil–based. **SERVES 2**

3 tablespoons (45 mL) low-fat sesame salad dressing

3 tablespoons (45 mL) fat-free mayonnaise (or 4 teaspoons/20 mL reduced-fat mayonnaise)

1 tablespoon (15 mL) miso paste

6 ounces (170 g) cooked skinless chicken breast, chopped or shredded

2 cups (500 mL) chopped fresh spinach

1 cup (250 mL) shredded carrots

1 cup (250 mL) sliced unpeeled English cucumber

2 low-carb high-fiber tortillas

1. In a medium bowl, stir together sesame dressing, mayonnaise, and miso.
2. Add chicken, spinach, carrots, and cucumber. Stir to mix well.
3. Warm tortillas (heat in a sauté pan over medium heat until pliable, or microwave for 30 seconds).
4. Divide salad mixture between tortillas. Fold or roll up.

### Nutritional Information (per serving)

Calories 280 • Carbs 36 grams • Protein 25 grams • Fat 10 grams • Fiber 17 grams

# Philly Cheesesteak Wrap

I promised you'd never feel deprived by the Body Reset Diet, and I meant it! This delicious wrap satisfies that cheesesteak craving without causing a post-cheesesteak food coma.  **SERVES 2**

Cooking oil spray

½ cup (125 mL) thinly sliced onion

¼ cup (60 mL) chopped mushrooms

½ cup (125 mL) thinly sliced green bell pepper

Salt and pepper

4 ounces (115 g) filet mignon, thinly sliced

2 low-carb high-fiber tortillas

2 tablespoons (30 mL) fat-free mayonnaise
   (or 1 tablespoon/15 mL reduced-fat mayonnaise)

½ cup (125 mL) fat-free mozzarella cheese

1. Heat a medium nonstick sauté pan over medium-high heat. Spray with cooking oil.
2. Add onions, mushrooms, and bell pepper; sauté until vegetables are soft. Remove from heat, season with salt and pepper, and set aside.
3. Return pan to heat. Add steak and cook just until cooked through, about 2 minutes. Transfer steak to a cutting board and chop.
4. Warm tortillas (heat in the wiped sauté pan over medium heat until pliable, or microwave for 30 seconds).
5. Spread tortillas with mayonnaise and top with beef, veggies, and cheese. Fold or roll up.

---

**Nutritional Information (per serving)**

Calories 276  •  Carbs 31 grams  •  Protein 29 grams  •  Fat 9 grams  •  Fiber 13 grams

# Shrimp Po'boy Wrap

This wrap was inspired by the fare of New Orleans, home to some of the best restaurants in North America.
**SERVES 2**

1 teaspoon (5 mL) olive oil

12 medium shrimp, peeled and deveined

1 teaspoon (5 mL) Cajun seasoning

Salt and pepper

½ cup (125 mL) canned white beans, drained and rinsed

½ cup (125 mL) fat-free hummus

2 low-carb high-fiber tortillas

2 cups (500 mL) shredded romaine lettuce

4 slices medium plum tomato

1. Heat a medium nonstick sauté pan over medium-high heat. Add oil.
2. Season shrimp with half of the Cajun seasoning and salt and pepper. Add to pan; sauté until cooked through, 3 to 4 minutes per side. Remove from pan and set aside.
3. In a small bowl, stir together beans, hummus, and remaining Cajun seasoning.
4. Warm tortillas (heat in a sauté pan over medium heat until pliable, or microwave for 30 seconds).
5. Spread tortillas with hummus mixture, then top with lettuce, tomato, and shrimp. Fold or roll up.

**Nutritional Information (per serving)**

Calories 289 • Carbs 46 grams • Protein 25 grams • Fat 6 grams • Fiber 20 grams

# Spicy Lentil Burger

This vegetarian burger is a must for you Sriracha fanatics out there.   **SERVES 2**

Cooking oil spray

½ cup (125 mL) chopped onions

1 cup (250 mL) cooked lentils

¾ cup (175 mL) canned chickpeas, drained and rinsed

2 tablespoons (30 mL) dry bread crumbs

1 teaspoon (5 mL) Worcestershire sauce

1 teaspoon (5 mL) Sriracha sauce

Salt and pepper

2 high-fiber hamburger buns

1. Heat a medium nonstick sauté pan over medium-high heat. Spray with cooking oil.
2. Add onions; sauté until soft, about 4 minutes.
3. In a food processor, combine onions, lentils, chickpeas, bread crumbs, Worcestershire sauce, and Sriracha sauce. Pulse until blended.
4. Heat a grill or nonstick sauté pan on medium-high heat. Spray with cooking oil.
5. Divide lentil mixture in half and shape by hand into 2 patties. Season with salt and pepper.
6. Grill patties, turning once, until firm, 5 to 7 minutes per side.
7. Shortly before patties are ready, place buns on grill to warm.
8. Serve burgers on warm buns.

| Nutritional Information (per serving) |
| --- |

Calories 380   •   Carbs 75 grams   •   Protein 20 grams   •   Fat 4 grams   •   Fiber 18 grams

# Spicy Black Bean Beet Burger

Store-bought veggie patties don't come anywhere close to this burger, and the reddish purple hue makes it interesting for kids! Instead of raw beets, you can use cooked or canned.   **SERVES 2**

Cooking oil spray

2 small beets, peeled and finely chopped

½ cup (125 mL) chopped onion

2 cloves garlic, chopped (or more if preferred)

1 cup (250 mL) canned black beans, drained and rinsed

1 tablespoon (15 mL) finely chopped canned chipotle chilies in adobo sauce (or 1 teaspoon/5 mL dried chipotle chili)

1 tablespoon (15 mL) Worcestershire sauce

1 tablespoon (15 mL) cider vinegar or other vinegar

Salt and pepper

¼ cup (60 mL) whole wheat flour

2 high-fiber hamburger buns

2 tablespoons (30 mL) fat-free mayonnaise (or 1 tablespoon/15 mL reduced-fat mayonnaise)

1. Heat a large nonstick sauté pan over medium-high heat. Spray with cooking oil.
2. Add beets, onions, and garlic; sauté until soft, about 6 minutes. Remove from heat.
3. In a food processor, combine beet mixture, beans, chipotles, Worcestershire sauce, and vinegar. Season with salt and pepper. Pulse just enough to combine and lightly chop the mixture (or combine in a large bowl and mix thoroughly by hand, keeping it chunky).
4. Transfer mixture to a large bowl (if using food processor) and add flour; mix thoroughly.
5. Divide mixture in half and shape by hand into 2 patties. If mixture is too loose to hold together, add a pinch more flour.
6. Return pan to medium-high heat. Sear patties until brown on the bottom, about 6 minutes. Flip patties, cover, reduce heat to medium-low, and cook until cooked through, about 6 minutes.
7. Spread top half of each bun with mayo and place a patty on each bun.

| Nutritional Information (per serving) |
| :---: |

Calories 385  •  Carbs 75 grams  •  Protein 18 grams  •  Fat 7 grams  •  Fiber 23 grams

# Herbed Chicken Barley Burger

Flavored with herbs and balsamic vinegar, this is a very grown-up burger! **SERVES 2**

1 teaspoon (5 mL) olive oil

1 cup (250 mL) chopped onion

1 tablespoon (15 mL) balsamic vinegar

2 cloves garlic, chopped

½ cup (125 mL) cooked barley

½ cup (125 mL) canned white beans, drained and rinsed

3½ ounces (100 g) ground chicken breast

1 teaspoon (5 mL) fresh oregano (or ½ teaspoon/2 mL dried)

1 teaspoon (5 mL) thyme

Cooking oil spray

Salt and pepper

2 high-fiber hamburger buns

1. Heat a medium nonstick sauté pan over medium-high heat. Add olive oil.
2. Add onions; sauté for 3 minutes.
3. Stir in vinegar; cook, stirring occasionally, for another 3 minutes. Remove from heat.
4. In a food processor, combine onions, garlic, barley, beans, chicken, oregano, and thyme. Pulse just until combined.
5. Heat grill or nonstick sauté pan on medium-high heat. Spray with cooking oil.
6. Divide chicken mixture in half and shape by hand into 2 patties. Season with salt and pepper.
7. Grill patties, turning once, until cooked through, about 5 minutes per side or until internal temperature reaches 165°F (74°C).
8. Shortly before patties are ready, place buns on grill to warm.
9. Serve burgers on warm buns.

**Nutritional Information (per serving)**

Calories 372 • Carbs 59 grams • Protein 21 grams • Fat 9 grams • Fiber 12 grams

# Grilled Black Bean Turkey Burger

If you like a good burger, then you'll love this healthy version made with ground turkey breast and black beans and packed with fiber and protein.  **SERVES 2**

7 ounces (200 g) ground turkey breast

¼ cup (60 mL) black beans, drained and rinsed, mashed lightly

2 tablespoons (30 mL) dry bread crumbs

1 tablespoon (15 mL) grated reduced-fat Parmesan cheese

1 tablespoon (15 mL) Worcestershire sauce

Salt and pepper

Cooking oil spray

2 high-fiber hamburger buns

2 teaspoons (10 mL) mustard

2 large romaine lettuce leaves

4 slices medium tomato

1. In a medium bowl, combine turkey, beans, bread crumbs, Parmesan, and Worcestershire sauce. Mix with your hands until combined. Season with salt and pepper. Shape into 2 patties.
2. Heat a medium nonstick sauté pan over medium-high heat. Spray with cooking oil.
3. Sear burgers on both sides, covered and turning once, until completely cooked through, about 4 minutes per side or until internal temperature reaches 165°F (74°C).
4. Spread mustard on each bun. Assemble burgers with lettuce and tomato.

## Nutritional Information (per serving)

Calories 325  •  Carbs 39 grams  •  Protein 23 grams  •  Fat 10 grams  •  Fiber 13 grams

# Turkey Bacon Burger

I love turkey bacon. I have this sandwich probably once a week.  **SERVES 2**

5 ounces (140 g) ground turkey breast

1 tablespoon (15 mL) Worcestershire sauce

2 teaspoons (10 mL) hot sauce (optional)

½ teaspoon (2 mL) dried thyme

½ teaspoon (2 mL) paprika

½ teaspoon (2 mL) garlic powder

2 slices turkey bacon, chopped

Salt and pepper

Cooking oil spray

2 slices low-fat cheese, such as Cheddar, or fat-free cheese singles

2 high-fiber hamburger buns

2 large romaine lettuce leaves

4 slices medium tomato

4 spears dill pickle

1. In a food processor, combine ground turkey, Worcestershire sauce, hot sauce (if using), thyme, paprika, and garlic powder. Pulse until well mixed. Add turkey bacon; pulse to blend.
2. Divide mixture in half and shape by hand into 2 patties. Season with salt and pepper.
3. Heat a medium nonstick sauté pan over medium-high heat. Spray with cooking oil.
4. Cook burgers, turning once, until browned and cooked through, about 5 minutes per side or until internal temperature reaches 165°F (74°C). In the last few minutes of cooking, top burgers with cheese and cover with lid.
5. Warm buns just before serving.
6. Serve burgers on buns topped with lettuce and tomato, with pickles on the side.

**Nutritional Information (per serving)**

Calories 367 • Carbs 24 grams • Protein 24 grams • Fat 8 grams • Fiber 8 grams

# Southwestern Turkey Burger

I always keep a Mexican-style corn blend (with bell peppers and jalapeño) in my freezer so that I can whip up this tasty burger in no time. **SERVES 4**

12 ounces (340 g) ground turkey breast

1 cup (250 mL) canned white beans, drained and rinsed, mashed lightly

1 cup (250 mL) fresh or thawed frozen corn kernels

½ cup (125 mL) diced red bell pepper

¼ cup (60 mL) chopped fresh cilantro

1 tablespoon (15 mL) taco seasoning mix, chili powder, or other spicy seasoning

Juice of 1 lime

Salt and pepper

Cooking oil spray

4 slices low-fat cheese, such as Cheddar, or fat-free cheese singles

4 high-fiber hamburger buns

¼ cup (60 mL) fat-free salsa

Hot sauce (optional)

1. In a large bowl, combine ground turkey, beans, corn, bell pepper, cilantro, taco seasoning, and lime juice. Season with salt and pepper. Mix by hand.
2. Divide mixture in 4 and shape by hand into 4 patties.
3. Heat a large nonstick sauté pan over medium-high heat. Spray with cooking oil.
4. Cook patties, turning once, until browned and cooked through, about 5 minutes per side or until internal temperature reaches 165°F (74°C). Top with cheese during last 2 minutes of cooking.
5. Warm buns just before serving.
6. Top buns with burgers. Top with salsa and hot sauce, if desired.

### Nutritional Information (per serving)

Calories 315 • Carbs 40 grams • Protein 37 grams • Fat 4 grams • Fiber 11 grams

# SOUPS AND STEWS

# Vegetable Barley Soup

Using tempeh in this classic soup adds major protein but keeps it vegetarian. **SERVES 4**

1 teaspoon (5 mL) olive oil

1 cup (250 mL) chopped onion

1 cup (250 mL) chopped carrots

3 cloves garlic, minced

4 cups (1 L) chopped Swiss chard

1 cup (250 mL) crumbled or chopped tempeh

1 can (14 ounces/398 mL) diced tomatoes

1 cup (250 mL) canned chickpeas, drained and rinsed

6 cups (1.5 L) fat-free vegetable broth

1 tablespoon (15 mL) dried or chopped fresh oregano

2 cups (500 mL) cooked pearl barley

Salt and pepper

1. Heat a soup pot over medium-high heat. Add olive oil.
2. Add onions, carrots, and garlic; sauté until soft, about 6 minutes.
3. Stir in chard and tempeh; sauté until chard is wilted.
4. Stir in tomatoes, chickpeas, vegetable broth, and oregano. Bring to a boil, reduce heat, and simmer for 20 minutes.
5. Stir in barley and heat through. Season with salt and pepper.

### Nutritional Information (per serving)

Calories 366 • Carbs 60 grams • Protein 20 grams • Fat 7 grams • Fiber 12 grams

# Spiced Lentil and Spinach Soup

Say goodbye to pricey canned soups. This soup tastes savory and delicious, and the olives satisfy your "salt tooth." **SERVES 4**

1 tablespoon (15 mL) olive oil

1 cup (250 mL) chopped onion

3 cloves garlic, minced

20 cups (5 L) fresh spinach (1¼ pounds/565 g), chopped

2 cans (14 ounces/398 mL each) diced tomatoes

8 cups (2 L) fat-free vegetable broth

1 tablespoon (15 mL) smoked paprika

1 teaspoon (5 mL) fresh or dried thyme

2 tablespoons (30 mL) Worcestershire sauce

2½ cups (625 mL) cooked lentils

¼ cup (60 mL) chopped pitted green olives

Salt and pepper

1. Heat a soup pot over medium-high heat. Add olive oil.
2. Add onions and garlic; sauté for 1 minute.
3. Add spinach; cook, stirring often, until spinach is wilted.
4. Add tomatoes and broth, stirring to scrape up any browned bits.
5. Stir in paprika, thyme, and Worcestershire sauce. Bring to a boil, reduce heat, and simmer for 20 minutes.
6. Stir in lentils and olives; heat through. Season with salt and pepper.

## Nutritional Information (per serving)

**Calories 357 • Carbs 52 grams • Protein 22 grams • Fat 9 grams • Fiber 17 grams**

# Broccoli White Bean Soup

The simplicity—and deliciousness—of this recipe will have you coming back to it over and over again.

**SERVES 2**

1¼ cups (300 mL) canned cannellini beans, drained and rinsed

4 cups (1 L) fat-free vegetable broth

1 tablespoon (15 mL) olive oil

½ cup (125 mL) chopped onion

2 cloves garlic, chopped

Chopped fresh rosemary and smoked paprika to taste (optional)

3 cups (750 mL) chopped broccoli florets

1 teaspoon (5 mL) dried thyme

Salt and pepper

¼ cup (60 mL) grated reduced-fat Parmesan cheese.

1. Purée beans with broth in a blender. Set aside.
2. Heat a large saucepan over medium-high heat. Add olive oil.
3. Add onions and garlic; sauté until soft.
4. Stir in rosemary and paprika (if using). Add broccoli; sauté for 2 to 3 minutes.
5. Stir in puréed beans and thyme. Cover, reduce heat to low, and simmer until reduced to desired thickness, 12 to 15 minutes.
6. Season with salt and pepper. Serve topped with Parmesan cheese.

**Nutritional Information (per serving)**

Calories 328 • Carbs 47 grams • Protein 17 grams • Fat 10 grams • Fiber 13 grams

# Spicy Corn Chowder with Edamame

Edamame, or fresh soybeans, are a delicious, versatile way to add protein to a vegetarian soup.
**SERVES 5**

2 cups (500 mL) canned white beans, drained and rinsed

8 cups (2 L) fat-free vegetable broth

Cooking oil spray

1 tablespoon (15 mL) light butter

1 medium onion, chopped

¾ cup (175 mL) chopped green bell pepper

¾ cup (175 mL) chopped red bell pepper

Salt and pepper

3 cups (750 mL) fresh or thawed frozen corn kernels

1 cup (250 mL) canned or thawed frozen shelled edamame

1 tablespoon (15 mL) chopped fresh or dried tarragon

1. Purée beans with 1 cup (250 mL) of the broth in a blender. Set aside.
2. Heat a soup pot over medium-high heat. Spray with cooking oil and add butter.
3. Add onions and bell peppers; season with salt and pepper. Sauté until soft, about 6 minutes.
4. Stir in corn and edamame; sauté until corn begins to lightly brown, about 5 minutes.
5. Add puréed beans, tarragon, and remaining 7 cups (1.75 L) broth; stir to combine.
6. Bring to a boil. Reduce heat and simmer for 20 minutes. Season with salt and pepper.

**Nutritional Information (per serving)**

Calories 374 • Carbs 67 grams • Protein 19 grams • Fat 5 grams • Fiber 12 grams

# Manhattan Style Fresh Salmon Chowder

Because fresh clams can be hard to come by depending on where you live and the season, I love to use heart-healthy salmon in this satisfying chowder.   **SERVES 4**

Cooking oil spray

2 slices turkey bacon, diced

4 cups (1 L) diced unpeeled potatoes (any kind)

1 cup (250 mL) chopped onion

1 cup (250 mL) diced red bell pepper

2 tablespoons (30 mL) tomato paste

1¼ cups (300 mL) canned diced tomatoes

4 cups (1 L) fat-free chicken broth

9 ounces (255 g) skinless salmon fillet, cut in bite-size pieces

1½ cups (375 mL) frozen corn kernels

2 tablespoons (30 mL) chopped fresh tarragon

Salt and pepper

1. Heat a soup pot over medium heat. Spray with cooking oil.
2. Add bacon; cook until crisp. Remove and set aside.
3. Add potatoes, onions, and bell pepper; cook, stirring often, until beginning to brown, about 6 minutes.
4. Add tomato paste and stir to coat vegetables.
5. Stir in tomatoes and broth. Bring to a boil.
6. Stir in salmon, corn, and tarragon. Reduce heat and simmer, uncovered, until broth has thickened and salmon is cooked through, about 30 minutes.
7. Season with salt and pepper. Serve garnished with the bacon.

---

**Nutritional Information (per serving)**

Calories 341  •  Carbs 52 grams  •  Protein 24 grams  •  Fat 6 grams  •  Fiber 8 grams

# Chinese Tofu and Greens Soup

The soup from your local Chinese delivery place won't hold a candle to this more authentic version, loaded with fresh greens and antioxidant powerhouse mushrooms.  **SERVES 4**

1 tablespoon (15 mL) sesame or canola oil

3 cloves garlic, chopped

¼ cup (60 mL) chopped peeled fresh ginger

8 ounces (225 g) low-fat extra-firm tofu, cubed

30 cups (7 L) fresh baby spinach
(2 pounds/900 g), chopped

4 cups (1 L) shredded or chopped napa
cabbage

4 cups (1 L) shredded or chopped bok choy

2 cups (500 mL) chopped shiitake mushrooms

2 cups (500 mL) canned or thawed frozen
shelled edamame

8 cups (2 L) fat-free vegetable broth

2 tablespoons (30 mL) low-sodium soy sauce

1 tablespoon (15 mL) fish sauce

Salt and pepper

1 cup (250 mL) chopped green onions

¼ cup (60 mL) chopped fresh cilantro

1. Heat a soup pot over medium-high heat. Add half of the sesame oil.
2. Add garlic and ginger; sauté until fragrant, about 30 seconds.
3. Add tofu; sauté until tofu begins to brown and crisp, about 5 minutes. Transfer mixture to a bowl.
4. Add remaining oil to pot. Working in batches, add spinach, cabbage, and bok choy, cooking until wilted, about 3 minutes per batch. Transfer to another bowl.
5. Add mushrooms and edamame to pot; cook, stirring often, until mushrooms are soft, about 5 minutes.
6. Add broth, soy sauce, and fish sauce. Bring to a boil. Reduce heat and simmer for 20 minutes.
7. Add greens to soup. Season with salt and pepper.
8. Divide among bowls and top with tofu mixture, green onions, and cilantro.

| Nutritional Information (per serving) |
| --- |

**Calories 325** • **Carbs 40 grams** • **Protein 27 grams** • **Fat 8 grams** • **Fiber 11 grams**

# Hearty Chicken and Vegetable Soup

Here's a classic recipe that I've redesigned, loading it with nutrients and without excess sodium or chemical preservatives.  **SERVES 4**

4 teaspoons (20 mL) olive oil

1 cup (250 mL) chopped onion

8 ounces (225 g) skinless chicken breast, chopped in small pieces or cut crosswise in ½-inch (1 cm) strips

Salt and pepper

2 cups (500 mL) chopped carrots

1 cup (250 mL) chopped celery

4 cups (1 L) chopped Swiss chard

8 cups (2 L) fat-free chicken broth

1 cup (250 mL) pearl barley

1 tablespoon (15 mL) chopped fresh parsley

1 tablespoon (15 mL) chopped fresh thyme

1. Heat a soup pot over medium-high heat. Add olive oil.
2. Add onions and chicken; season with salt and pepper. Sauté until chicken is cooked through, about 7 minutes.
3. Add carrots and celery; sauté until carrots are soft, about 5 minutes.
4. Stir in chard; cook until wilted, about 3 minutes.
5. Add broth. Bring to a boil.
6. Stir in barley, parsley, and thyme. Reduce heat to low, cover, and simmer until barley is tender, at least 45 minutes. Add water if necessary. Season with salt and pepper.

### Nutritional Information (per serving)

Calories 388  •  Carbs 60 grams  •  Protein 25 grams  •  Fat 7 grams  •  Fiber 15 grams

# Tuscan Kale and Chicken Soup

This soup is an ode to Tuscan cuisine, which is characterized by its fresh, simple preparations that let the ingredients shine without smothering them in heavy sauces.  **SERVES 2**

Cooking oil spray

½ cup (125 mL) chopped onion

½ cup (125 mL) chopped carrots

½ cup (125 mL) chopped celery

½ cup (125 mL) chopped fennel

4 cups (1 L) chopped kale

2 cloves garlic, chopped

1 teaspoon (5 mL) chopped fresh thyme

1 teaspoon (5 mL) dried oregano

3 ounces (85 g) skinless chicken breast, cooked and shredded

⅔ cup (150 mL) canned cannellini beans, drained and rinsed

4 cups (1 L) fat-free vegetable broth

Salt and pepper

1. Heat a medium saucepan over medium-high heat. Spray with cooking oil.
2. Add onions, carrots, celery, and fennel; sauté until vegetables are almost soft, about 4 minutes.
3. Stir in kale and garlic; cook until kale has wilted, about 5 minutes.
4. Stir in thyme, oregano, chicken, beans, and broth; season with salt and pepper. Simmer for 15 minutes.

**Nutritional Information (per serving)**

Calories 323  •  Carbs 48 grams  •  Protein 27 grams  •  Fat 5 grams  •  Fiber 10 grams

# Sweet Potato, Chicken, and Kale Soup

I love using sweet potatoes in place of regular white potatoes. They have more vitamin C, vitamin A, and all-important fiber.  **SERVES 2**

Cooking oil spray

¾ cup (175 mL) chopped leeks

1 clove garlic, minced

3 cups (750 mL) diced peeled sweet potato (about 2 medium)

4 cups (1 L) fat-free chicken broth

2 cups (500 mL) water

8 ounces (225 g) skinless chicken breast, chopped in small pieces

2 tablespoons (30 mL) almond butter

8 cups (2 L) chopped kale

1 teaspoon (5 mL) minced peeled fresh ginger

Hot pepper flakes (optional)

Salt and pepper

1. Heat a soup pot over medium-high heat. Spray with cooking oil.
2. Add leeks; sauté until they begin to soften, about 5 minutes.
3. Add garlic; sauté for 1 minute.
4. Add sweet potatoes, broth, and water. Bring to a boil.
5. Stir in chicken; reduce heat and simmer until chicken is cooked through, about 10 minutes.
6. Transfer 1 cup (250 mL) of the hot soup to a small bowl and whisk in almond butter. Stir mixture into soup.
7. Stir in kale, ginger, and hot pepper flakes (if using); simmer until kale is soft, about 10 minutes. Season with salt and pepper.

**Nutritional Information (per serving)**

Calories 317  •  Carbs 44 grams  •  Protein 21 grams  •  Fat 9 grams  •  Fiber 10 grams

# Turkey Bacon, Bean, and Tomato Soup

This rib-sticking soup is packed with flavor, leaving you completely satisfied.  **SERVES 2**

Cooking oil spray

4 slices turkey bacon

2 large celery ribs, diced

½ cup (125 mL) diced onion

2 small tomatoes, diced

6 tablespoons (90 mL) tomato paste

1 teaspoon (5 mL) dried Italian herb seasoning

Chopped fresh thyme and rosemary to taste (optional)

2 cups (500 mL) assorted canned beans (such as lima, kidney, black, white), drained and rinsed

4 cups (1 L) fat-free chicken broth

Salt and pepper

1. Heat a medium saucepan over medium-high heat. Spray with cooking oil.
2. Add bacon, celery, and onions; sauté until bacon is browned and vegetables are soft.
3. Stir in tomatoes, tomato paste, Italian seasoning, fresh herbs, beans, and broth. Reduce heat to low and simmer for at least 20 minutes. Season with salt and pepper.

**Nutritional Information (per serving)**

Calories 336  •  Carbs 48 grams  •  Protein 31 grams  •  Fat 5 grams  •  Fiber 15 grams

# Cauliflower Soup with Bacon-Cheddar Topping

Kids (and grown-ups) love this soup and will never suspect that cauliflower is at its base.  **SERVES 3**

3 slices turkey bacon, chopped

Cooking oil spray

½ cup (125 mL) chopped onion

4 celery ribs, chopped

1 clove garlic, chopped

Salt and pepper

2 medium heads cauliflower, chopped

1 cup (250 mL) water

2 cups (500 mL) fat-free chicken broth

2 cups (500 mL) 2% milk

1¼ cups (300 mL) shredded low-fat
   Cheddar cheese

1 green onion, chopped (optional)

1. Sauté bacon in a soup pot until crisp. Drain on paper towels. Set aside.
2. Spray pot with cooking oil. Add onions, celery, and garlic; season with salt and pepper. Cook, stirring often, until vegetables begin to soften, 5 to 6 minutes.
3. Add cauliflower and water. Cover and steam until cauliflower is tender, about 5 minutes.
4. Add broth and milk. Bring to a boil.
5. Working in batches if needed, in a blender, blend soup until smooth. Return soup to pot.
6. Simmer until soup is the desired thickness. Season with salt and pepper if needed.
7. Remove from heat and stir in half of the cheese.
8. Divide soup among bowls. Top with remaining cheese, bacon, and green onions (if using).

**Nutritional Information (per serving)**

Calories 307  •  Carbs 36 grams  •  Protein 28 grams  •  Fat 7 grams  •  Fiber 12 grams

# Italian Sausage and Kale Soup

This soup is my cross between *pasta e fagioli* and Italian Wedding Soup. I prefer kale instead of spinach because kale holds up really well in soups, even after freezing and reheating. **SERVES 4**

Cooking oil spray

½ cup (125 mL) chopped onion

3 cloves garlic, chopped

2 Italian sausages (chicken and pork, or 3 chicken), cooked, casings removed, shredded or finely chopped

8 cups (2 L) chopped kale

Salt and pepper

1 can (14 ounces/398 mL) diced tomatoes

2 cups (500 mL) canned white beans, drained and rinsed

1 tablespoon (15 mL) dried Italian herb seasoning

6 cups (1.5 L) fat-free vegetable broth

1. Heat a soup pot over medium-high heat. Spray with cooking oil.
2. Add onions and garlic. Sauté until onions are soft, about 3 minutes.
3. Stir in sausage. Stir in kale; cook until wilted, about 4 minutes. Season with salt and pepper.
4. Add tomatoes, beans, Italian seasoning, and broth. Bring to a boil, reduce heat, and simmer for 15 minutes. Season with salt and pepper.

**Nutritional Information (per serving)**

Calories 375 • Carbs 53 grams • Protein 26 grams • Fat 9 grams • Fiber 12 grams

# White Bean Chicken Chili

With 30 grams of protein and 14 grams of fiber per serving, this hearty chili will fill you up and keep you full for hours. **SERVES 2**

Cooking oil spray

½ cup (125 mL) finely chopped onion

1 clove garlic, finely chopped

2 cups (500 mL) chopped Swiss chard

1½ teaspoons (7 mL) ground cumin

1 teaspoon (5 mL) fennel seeds

1 teaspoon (5 mL) chili powder

1 teaspoon (5 mL) hot pepper flakes

1 bay leaf

Salt and pepper

4 ounces (115 g) skinless chicken breast, cooked and shredded

1½ cups (375 mL) canned cannellini beans, drained and rinsed

1 cup (250 mL) fresh corn kernels

½ cup (125 mL) canned chopped green chilies

4 cups (1 L) fat-free chicken broth

1 teaspoon (5 mL) Worcestershire sauce

1. Heat a soup pot over medium-high heat. Spray with cooking oil.
2. Add onions; sauté until soft, about 5 minutes.
3. Add garlic and chard; cook, stirring, until chard has wilted, about 4 minutes.
4. Stir in cumin, fennel seeds, chili powder, hot pepper flakes, and bay leaf. Season with salt and pepper.
5. Add chicken, beans, corn, and green chilies; stir to combine. Add broth and Worcestershire sauce.
6. Bring to a boil. Cover, reduce heat to low, and simmer until broth thickens, 20 to 30 minutes.

### Nutritional Information (per serving)

Calories 372 • Carbs 56 grams • Protein 30 grams • Fat 5 grams • Fiber 14 grams

# BBQ Chicken Chili

I like to double or triple this recipe and freeze the extra for those days when my wife and I don't have even five minutes to throw some dinner together. **SERVES 5**

1 tablespoon (15 mL) olive or other oil

1 cup (250 mL) chopped onions

3 cloves garlic, minced

8 ounces (225 g) ground chicken breast

1 cup (250 mL) chopped fresh peppers (such as Anaheim, Hatch, bell, jalapeño)

2 cans (14 ounces/398 mL each) beans (such as black, pinto, kidney), drained and rinsed

1 can (14 ounces/398 mL) diced tomatoes

1 can (14 ounces/398 mL) puréed tomatoes

2 tablespoons (30 mL) chili powder

1 tablespoon (15 mL) ground cumin

2 tablespoons (30 mL) Worcestershire sauce

2 tablespoons (30 mL) cider vinegar or other vinegar

1 teaspoon (5 mL) stevia or sweetener of your choice

Shredded fat-free cheese and chopped green onions, for garnish

1. Heat a soup pot over medium-high heat. Add olive oil.
2. Add onions, garlic, and chicken; sauté until chicken is cooked through and lightly colored, about 7 minutes.
3. Add peppers; sauté until soft, about 4 minutes.
4. Add beans, diced tomatoes, puréed tomatoes, chili powder, cumin, Worcestershire sauce, vinegar, and stevia; stir to combine.
5. Bring to a boil, reduce heat, and simmer, uncovered, for 20 to 45 minutes. The longer it cooks, the more the flavor develops.
6. Divide among bowls and top with cheese and green onions, if desired.

**Nutritional Information (per serving)**

Calories 348 • Carbs 54 grams • Protein 28 grams • Fat 4 grams • Fiber 14 grams

# Hearty Beef Stew

Although I now call Los Angeles home, I'll never forget how truly cold it gets in my hometown of Toronto. This stew is perfect for those really chilly days when you need to be warmed from the inside out.
**SERVES 4**

1 tablespoon (15 mL) extra-virgin olive oil

12 ounces (340 g) lean beef chuck, trimmed of excess fat and cut in bite-size pieces

Salt and pepper

Cooking oil spray

1½ cups (375 mL) cubed peeled sweet potato

1¼ cups (300 mL) carrots cut in bite-size pieces

1 cup (250 mL) mushrooms, halved if large

½ cup (125 mL) finely chopped onion

½ cup (125 mL) finely chopped celery

1 clove garlic, finely chopped

1½ cups (375 mL) canned chickpeas, drained and rinsed

1 teaspoon (5 mL) fresh thyme

1 bay leaf

4 cups (1 L) fat-free beef broth

2 tablespoons (30 mL) Worcestershire sauce

1 tablespoon (15 mL) tomato paste

1 cup (250 mL) thawed frozen peas

1. Heat olive oil in a large pot over high heat. Season beef with salt and pepper.
2. Working in batches so you don't crowd the pot, sauté beef until browned and crusty all over, about 4 minutes per side. Remove from pot as cooked and set aside.
3. Spray pot with cooking oil. Add sweet potatoes, carrots, mushrooms, onions, celery, and garlic; sauté until vegetables are soft and beginning to brown, about 8 minutes.
4. Return beef and any juices to pot. Add chickpeas, thyme, and bay leaf.
5. Add 1 cup (250 mL) of the broth. Stir, scraping browned bits from bottom and sides of pan.
6. Add remaining 3 cups (750 mL) broth, Worcestershire sauce, and tomato paste; stir to combine. Reduce heat, cover, and simmer until stew reaches desired consistency, at least 20 minutes.
7. Stir in peas. Season with salt and pepper if needed.

**Nutritional Information (per serving)**

Calories 385 • Carbs 47 grams • Protein 26 grams • Fat 10 grams • Fiber 9 grams

# STIR-FRIES AND SAUTÉS

# Ginger and Garlic Tofu Stir-Fry

This is a simple recipe with clean flavors. If I'm in the mood for a little more heat, I throw some hot pepper flakes in the pan. **SERVES 4**

Cooking oil spray

1/4 cup (60 mL) chopped onion

1/4 cup (60 mL) minced peeled fresh ginger

3 cloves garlic, minced

2 cups (500 mL) low-fat firm tofu

2 cups (500 mL) diced peeled sweet potato

1 bunch broccolini or Chinese broccoli, chopped

4 cups (1 L) shredded cabbage (any kind)

1/2 cup (125 mL) water

Salt

3 cups (750 mL) cooked quinoa

1. Heat a wok or large nonstick sauté pan over high heat. Spray with cooking oil.
2. Add onions, ginger, and garlic; stir-fry until fragrant, about 1 minute.
3. Add tofu; stir-fry until tofu begins to brown, about 4 minutes. Transfer tofu mixture to a bowl.
4. Spray pan again. Add sweet potatoes; stir-fry until they begin to caramelize, about 5 minutes.
5. Add broccolini and cabbage; stir-fry until they begin to soften, 5 to 8 minutes.
6. Add water; cover and steam for 4 minutes.
7. Stir in tofu mixture and heat through. Season to taste with salt.
8. Place 3/4 cup (175 mL) quinoa in each of 4 large dishes. Top with stir-fry.

## Nutritional Information (per serving)

Calories 385 • Carbs 57 grams • Protein 22 grams • Fat 9 grams • Fiber 10 grams

# Chicken Quinoa Stir-Fry

I enjoy this stir-fry on its own, but for a little change of pace it's great spooned into Bibb lettuce cups.
**SERVES 2**

Cooking oil spray

1 tablespoon (15 mL) grated or finely chopped
    peeled fresh ginger

1 clove garlic, finely chopped

5 ounces (140 g) skinless chicken breast,
    chopped in small pieces

1 cup (250 mL) thinly sliced red bell pepper

1 cup (250 mL) frozen peas

½ cup (125 mL) thinly sliced or chopped
    red cabbage

Salt and pepper

2 large eggs, beaten

1½ cups (375 mL) cooked quinoa

2 tablespoons (30 mL) low-sodium
    soy sauce

Juice of 1 lime

¼ cup (60 mL) chopped fresh cilantro

2 large green onions, finely chopped

1. Heat a wok or large nonstick sauté pan over high heat. Spray with cooking oil.
2. Add ginger, garlic, and chicken; stir-fry until chicken begins to brown, about 5 minutes, making sure not to let the garlic burn.
3. Add red pepper, peas, and cabbage; season with salt and pepper. Stir-fry for another 4 minutes.
4. Push chicken mixture to edges of pan. Add eggs to middle of pan. Scramble the eggs, then stir in chicken mixture.
5. Add quinoa, soy sauce, and lime juice; stir to combine. Cook for another 2 to 3 minutes.
6. Divide stir-fry between 2 bowls. Top with cilantro and green onions.

**Nutritional Information (per serving)**

Calories 386 • Carbs 52 grams • Protein 31 grams • Fat 6 grams • Fiber 10 grams

# Tofu Chickpea Curry

This vegetarian sauté is inspired by the hearty meat-free meals common in South Asian cuisine.

**SERVES 4**

1 teaspoon (5 mL) canola oil

1 cup (250 mL) chopped onion

¼ cup (60 mL) minced peeled fresh ginger

1 pound (450 g) low-fat firm tofu, cubed

2 cups (500 mL) cubed peeled sweet potato

2 cups (500 mL) chopped carrots

2 cups (500 mL) canned chickpeas, drained and rinsed

¼ cup (60 mL) curry powder

¼ cup (60 mL) water

20 cups (5 L) fresh spinach (1¼ pounds/565 g), chopped

1 cup (250 mL) thawed frozen peas

Salt and pepper

Chopped fresh cilantro, for garnish

1. Heat a wok or large nonstick sauté pan over medium-high heat. Add oil.
2. Add onions and ginger; stir-fry for 1 minute.
3. Add tofu; stir-fry until tofu begins to brown and onions are soft, about 5 minutes.
4. Add sweet potatoes, carrots, and chickpeas; stir-fry for 8 minutes.
5. Stir in curry powder. Stir in water, cover, and cook for 5 minutes.
6. Stir in spinach and peas; cook, uncovered, until spinach is wilted. Season with salt and pepper.
7. Divide stir-fry among 4 dishes. Top with fresh cilantro, if desired.

**Nutritional Information (per serving)**

Calories 374 • Carbs 64 grams • Protein 24 grams • Fat 5 grams • Fiber 16 grams

# Coconut Shrimp Curry

This is one of my absolute favorite stir-fries. It's rich and delicious and perfect any time of year.   **SERVES 4**

1 teaspoon (5 mL) coconut oil or any vegetable oil

2 cups (500 mL) diced purple, red, or other potato

1 cup (250 mL) chopped onion

1 cup (250 mL) diced bell pepper (any color)

12 ounces (340 g) shrimp, peeled and deveined

1 cup (250 mL) chopped tomato

2 tablespoons curry powder or to taste

1 can (14 ounces/398 mL) chickpeas, drained and rinsed

1 tablespoon (15 mL) fish sauce

4 cups (1 L) fat-free chicken broth

1 can (14 ounces/398 mL) light coconut milk

4 cups (1 L) chopped broccoli

¼ cup (60 mL) chopped fresh basil

Salt and pepper

1. Heat a soup pot over medium-high heat. Add oil.
2. Add potatoes, onions, and bell pepper; stir-fry for 4 minutes.
3. Stir in shrimp; stir-fry for about 4 minutes.
4. Add tomatoes; stir-fry for 2 minutes.
5. Stir in curry powder. Add chickpeas, fish sauce, broth, and coconut milk. Bring to a boil, reduce heat, and simmer for 15 minutes.
6. Stir in broccoli; simmer, stirring occasionally, until broccoli is just tender, about 10 minutes.
7. Stir in basil. Season with salt and pepper.

| Nutritional Information (per serving) |
| --- |

Calories 371  •  Carbs 46 grams  •  Protein 28 grams  •  Fat 9 grams  •  Fiber 10 grams

# Chicken, Cashew, and Veggie Stir-Fry

Next time you're craving Chinese food, skip the grease (and expense!) and whip up this delicious stir-fry in a matter of minutes.  **SERVES 4**

2 tablespoons (30 mL) cornstarch

½ cup (125 mL) fat-free chicken broth

6 ounces (170 g) skinless chicken breast, chopped

¼ cup (60 mL) sliced peeled fresh ginger

2 cloves garlic, chopped

2½ teaspoons (12 mL) grapeseed or other vegetable oil

Salt and pepper

4 cups (1 L) chopped or thinly sliced broccoli

3 cups (750 mL) sliced zucchini

1 cup (250 mL) sliced red bell pepper

2 tablespoons (30 mL) low-sodium soy sauce

1 teaspoon (5 mL) hoisin sauce

4 cups (1 L) cooked brown rice

5 raw cashews, chopped

1. In a small bowl, whisk together cornstarch and broth; set aside.
2. In a bowl, mix together chicken, ginger, and garlic.
3. Heat a wok or large nonstick sauté pan over medium heat. Add oil.
4. Add chicken; season with salt and pepper. Stir-fry until chicken is almost cooked through.
5. Add broccoli, zucchini, and bell pepper; stir-fry until vegetables are cooked through, 5 to 8 minutes.
6. Stir in soy sauce and hoisin sauce. Stir cornstarch mixture and add. Stir to evenly coat chicken and vegetables. The sauce will thicken immediately.
7. Serve stir-fry over brown rice, topped with cashews.

## Nutritional Information (per serving)

Calories 392  •  Carbs 68 grams  •  Protein 20 grams  •  Fat 5 grams  •  Fiber 10 grams

# BBQ Pork and Sweet Potatoes

This quick and easy stir-fry is perfect for your next dinner party.   **SERVES 4**

1 medium unpeeled pear, cored and chopped

1 medium unpeeled apple, cored and chopped

1 cup (250 mL) chopped onion

½ cup (125 mL) low-sodium soy sauce

1 teaspoon (5 mL) stevia or sweetener of your choice

5 cloves garlic, minced

¼ cup (60 mL) minced peeled fresh ginger

2 teaspoons (10 mL) sesame oil

8 ounces (225 g) pork tenderloin, sliced in thin medallions

2 medium sweet potatoes, peeled and diced

32 cups (7.6 L) fresh spinach (2 pounds/900 g)

Salt and pepper

Cooking oil spray

1. In a blender, combine pear, apple, onions, soy sauce, stevia, half the garlic, half the ginger, and 1 teaspoon (5 mL) of the sesame oil; blend until smooth. Set aside ¼ cup (60 mL) of the marinade. Pour remaining marinade over pork medallions in a shallow dish or resealable plastic bag; marinate at room temperature for at least 20 minutes or refrigerate overnight.

2. Heat a wok or large nonstick sauté pan over medium-high heat. Add remaining 1 teaspoon (5 mL) sesame oil.

3. Add remaining ginger and garlic; stir-fry until fragrant, about 1 minute.

4. Add sweet potatoes; stir-fry until beginning to brown, about 5 minutes. Transfer sweet potato mixture to a bowl and set aside, keeping warm.

5. Add spinach to pan; sauté for 5 minutes. Season with salt. Transfer to another bowl and set aside, keeping warm.

6. Remove pork from marinade, letting excess marinade drip off; discard marinade. Season pork with salt and pepper.

7. Wipe pan with paper towel and set over high heat. Spray with cooking oil.

8. Add pork and reserved marinade to pan; cook until pork is browned on each side and marinade has thickened, about 6 minutes.

9. Divide spinach among 4 plates. Top with pork medallions and serve with sweet potatoes.

| Nutritional Information (per serving) |
|---|

Calories 353   •   Carbs 43 grams   •   Protein 33 grams   •   Fat 9 grams   •   Fiber 10 grams

# Steak and Veggie Stir-Fry

When you're buying the sirloin for this recipe, have the meat counter trim and slice the steak for you. It saves time and money! **SERVES 2**

Cooking oil spray

5 ounces (140 g) sirloin steak, trimmed of excess fat and thinly sliced

Salt and pepper

2 teaspoons (10 mL) coconut oil

2 cloves garlic, chopped

½ cup (125 mL) chopped onion

10 cups (2.4 L) fresh spinach (1 pound/450 g), chopped

2 cups (500 mL) chopped cabbage (any kind)

1 cup (250 mL) chopped red bell pepper

1 cup (250 mL) shredded carrots

1 cup (250 mL) sliced sugar snap peas

¼ cup (60 mL) low-sodium soy sauce

Sesame seeds, for garnish

1. Heat a wok or large nonstick sauté pan over high heat. Spray with cooking oil.
2. Meanwhile, season beef with salt and pepper.
3. Sear beef on each side, about 3 minutes total. Transfer to a plate and set aside.
4. Return pan to medium-high heat. Add coconut oil.
5. Add garlic and onions; stir-fry until onions are soft, 3 to 4 minutes.
6. Add spinach, cabbage, bell pepper, carrots, and snap peas; sauté until vegetables begin to soften, 5 to 8 minutes.
7. Stir in soy sauce. Return beef and any accumulated juices to pan; stir to combine and heat through.
8. Divide between 2 plates and top with sesame seeds.

**Nutritional Information (per serving)**

Calories 318 • Carbs 34 grams • Protein 27 grams • Fat 10 grams • Fiber 13 grams

# Cold Thai Peanut Noodles

Shirataki noodles are a Japanese noodle made from yams. They are a low-calorie alternative to pasta. Look for them in the international or chilled section of your grocery store. **SERVES 2**

2 cups (500 mL) thinly shredded cabbage
  (any kind)

2 cups (500 mL) shredded carrot

1 cup (250 mL) thinly sliced red bell pepper

¼ cup (60 mL) chopped fresh cilantro

8 ounces (225 g) tofu shirataki noodles,
  drained and rinsed

6 ounces (170 g) cooked skinless chicken
  breast, shredded

Salt

½ medium avocado, peeled and diced

Chopped fresh mint and basil, for garnish

¼ cup (60 mL) chopped green onions

1½ teaspoons (7 mL) sesame seeds, for garnish

**DRESSING**

¼ cup (60 mL) low-sodium soy sauce

1 tablespoon (15 mL) minced peeled fresh
  ginger

2 teaspoons (10 mL) reduced-fat peanut butter

Juice of 2 limes

Sriracha sauce

1. For the dressing: In a large bowl, combine soy sauce, ginger, peanut butter, and lime juice; whisk until smooth. Whisk in Sriracha sauce to taste.
2. Add cabbage, carrots, bell pepper, cilantro, noodles, and chicken. Toss to coat with dressing. Season with salt.
3. Cover and refrigerate for at least 30 minutes before serving.
4. Serve topped with avocado. Garnish with chopped herbs, green onions, and sesame seeds, if desired.

| Nutritional Information (per serving) |
| --- |

Calories 339 • Carbs 34 grams • Protein 34 grams • Fat 9 grams • Fiber 11 grams

# Spicy Greens with Tempeh

Between the tempeh, the Swiss chard, and the kale, this vegetarian dish is loaded with iron, which many vegetarians lack in their diets.  **SERVES 2**

1 teaspoon (5 mL) olive oil

6 ounces (170 g) tempeh, diced or crumbled

1 cup (250 mL) chopped onion

4 cups (1 L) chopped kale

2 cloves garlic, chopped

2 tablespoons (30 mL) fennel seeds

2 tablespoons (30 mL) Worcestershire sauce

2 teaspoons (10 mL) hot pepper flakes

Salt and pepper

2 cups (500 mL) fat-free vegetable broth

4 cups (1 L) chopped Swiss chard

1. Heat a soup pot over medium heat. Add oil.
2. Add tempeh and onions; cook, stirring often, until tempeh has begun to crisp and onions are soft, about 5 minutes.
3. Add kale and garlic; cook, stirring often, until wilted.
4. Stir in fennel seeds, Worcestershire sauce, and hot pepper flakes. Season with salt and pepper. Add broth, scraping up any browned bits on bottom of pan.
5. Add chard; simmer until chard and kale are soft and liquid has reduced, 5 to 8 minutes.

### Nutritional Information (per serving)

Calories 341  •  Carbs 46 grams  •  Protein 22 grams  •  Fat 10 grams  •  Fiber 15 grams

# Pad Thai

As pad thai's popularity grew in North America, it seemed to get further from its roots as a fresh, fragrant dish full of fresh veggies and closer to pasta with peanut sauce. This version tastes like the original.
**SERVES 2**

Cooking oil spray

8 ounces (225 g) low-fat firm silken tofu

2 cups (500 mL) whole or chopped sugar snap peas

2 cups (500 mL) mung bean sprouts, washed

2 cups (500 mL) chopped bok choy

1 cup (250 mL) canned or thawed frozen shelled edamame

2 cups (500 mL) chopped broccoli stems and florets

½ cup (125 mL) water

4 ounces (115 g) rice noodles, cooked

¼ cup (60 mL) pad thai sauce

2 tablespoons (30 mL) chopped peanuts

Chopped fresh cilantro, basil, and/or mint

Lime wedges

1. Heat a wok or large nonstick sauté pan over high heat. Spray with cooking oil.
2. Add tofu; sauté until beginning to brown, about 5 minutes. Transfer to a plate and set aside.
3. Spray wok again. Add snap peas, bean sprouts, bok choy, and edamame; sauté until bok choy has wilted and snap peas are tender-crisp, about 5 minutes.
4. Add broccoli and water. Cover and steam for 2 minutes.
5. Return tofu to pan along with rice noodles and pad thai sauce; stir to combine. Heat through.
6. Divide between 2 large bowls. Top with peanuts and chopped herbs. Serve with lime wedges.

**Nutritional Information (per serving)**

Calories 386 • Carbs 47 grams • Protein 26 grams • Fat 11 grams • Fiber 10 grams

# Vegetable Bolognese

This is a great dish for when you're hosting vegetarians or if you're just not in the mood for meat.

**SERVES 4**

1½ teaspoons (7 mL) olive oil

¼ cup (60 mL) chopped red onion

2 cloves garlic, minced

½ cup (125 mL) diced carrot

1 cup (250 mL) crumbled, shredded, or
  diced tempeh

2 cups (500 mL) diced mushrooms

1 can (14 ounces/398 mL) artichoke hearts,
  drained and diced

Salt and pepper

3 cups (750 mL) canned diced tomatoes

1 cup (250 mL) tomato purée or sauce

2 tablespoons (30 mL) Worcestershire sauce

1 tablespoon (15 mL) fennel seeds

1 teaspoon (5 mL) hot pepper flakes

10 cups (2.4 L) fresh spinach (1 pound/450 g),
  chopped

8 ounces (225 g) whole-grain pasta, cooked

Chopped fresh basil, for garnish

1. Heat a soup pot over medium-high heat. Add olive oil.
2. Add onions; sauté until fragrant, about 1 minute.
3. Add garlic, carrots, and tempeh; cook, stirring occasionally, until onions and carrots are soft, about 4 minutes.
4. Add mushrooms and artichokes; season with salt and pepper. Sauté until mushrooms are tender, about 5 minutes.
5. Add diced tomatoes, tomato purée, Worcestershire sauce, fennel seeds, and hot pepper flakes; stir to combine. Bring to a boil, reduce heat, and simmer for 15 to 20 minutes. Stir in spinach during last 5 minutes of cooking. Season with salt and pepper.
6. Divide cooked pasta among 4 dishes. Spoon approximately 1½ cups (375 mL) sauce over each serving. (Alternatively, stir pasta into Bolognese and then divide.) Garnish with basil.

**Nutritional Information (per serving)**

Calories 395 • Carbs 74 grams • Protein 18 grams • Fat 6 grams • Fiber 11 grams

# Miso Cod with Spinach and Sweet Potatoes

Sweet potatoes and miso strike a perfect balance between sweet and savory in this nutritious dish. Look for aji-mirin, a sweet rice wine, in the Asian foods section of the supermarket.   **SERVES 2**

4 teaspoons (20 mL) white miso paste

1 tablespoon (15 mL) low-sodium soy sauce

1 tablespoon (15 mL) aji-mirin

2 skinless cod fillets (3 ounces/85 g each)

Cooking oil spray

2 cups (500 mL) sweet potato sliced ¼ inch (5 mm) thick

1 teaspoon (5 mL) canola oil

Salt and pepper

20 cups (5 L) fresh spinach (1¼ pounds/565 g)

¼ medium avocado, peeled and chopped in small pieces

Sesame seeds (optional)

1. In a small bowl, stir together miso, soy sauce, and mirin. Set aside 2 teaspoons (10 mL) of marinade for the potatoes.
2. Coat all sides of cod with marinade. Marinate, covered and refrigerated, for at least 20 minutes or overnight for maximum flavor.
3. Preheat oven to 400°F (200°C). Spray a baking sheet with cooking oil.
4. In a large bowl, toss sweet potatoes with canola oil, reserved marinade, and a pinch each of salt and pepper. Spread in a single layer on the baking sheet. Bake, turning once halfway through, until browned, about 15 minutes.
5. Meanwhile, heat both a small and a large nonstick sauté pan over medium-high heat. Spray both with cooking oil.
6. Add spinach to large sauté pan, working in batches if needed; cook until just wilted. Season with a pinch of salt.
7. Add cod to small sauté pan; cook, turning once, until browned on both sides and cooked through, about 4 minutes per side.
8. Divide spinach and sweet potatoes between 2 plates. Top with cod. Top sweet potatoes with avocado and sesame seeds (if using).

### Nutritional Information (per serving)

Calories 376  •  Carbs 53 grams  •  Protein 28 grams  •  Fat 8 grams  •  Fiber 12 grams

# Pan-Roasted Chicken with Fennel and Tomatoes

Cooking this chicken dinner makes me feel like I'm on *Top Chef*. The fennel and rapini turn it into a stunning meal fit for your most discerning guest.  **SERVES 2**

1½ teaspoons (7 mL) olive oil

¼ cup (60 mL) chopped red onion

2 cloves garlic, minced

2 cups (500 mL) chopped fennel

6 ounces (170 g) skinless chicken breast, thinly sliced crosswise

Salt and pepper

4 cups (1 L) halved cherry tomatoes

2 tablespoons (30 mL) Worcestershire sauce

2 tablespoons (30 mL) balsamic vinegar

2 cups (500 mL) chopped rapini

2 tablespoons (30 mL) crumbled soft goat cheese

1. Heat a large nonstick sauté pan over medium-high heat. Add olive oil.
2. Add onions and garlic; sauté until fragrant, about 1 minute.
3. Add fennel; sauté until soft, about 6 minutes. Transfer to a plate and set aside.
4. Return pan to heat. Add chicken; season with salt and pepper. Sauté until chicken begins to brown and is mostly cooked through, about 4 minutes. Transfer chicken to plate with fennel.
5. Return pan to heat. Add tomatoes; sauté until they begin to blister and pop. Stir in Worcestershire sauce and balsamic vinegar.
6. Stir in rapini, fennel, and chicken; season with salt and pepper. Cover, reduce heat, and simmer until flavors combine, about 10 minutes.
7. Serve topped with goat cheese.

| Nutritional Information (per serving) |
| --- |

Calories 315  •  Carbs 34 grams  •  Protein 30 grams  •  Fat 9 grams  •  Fiber 10 grams

# Lemon Caper Chicken and Artichokes with Fettuccine

I love this meal; it reminds me of chicken piccata (my father-in-law's favorite), but unlike the classic, it's not weighed down by a heavy flour-and-butter batter. **SERVES 2**

1 tablespoon (15 mL) olive oil

¼ cup (60 mL) chopped shallot or onion

6 ounces (170 g) skinless chicken breast, sliced horizontally into 2 thin fillets

Salt and pepper

2 tablespoons (30 mL) white wine (optional)

¼ cup (60 mL) fat-free chicken broth

2 tablespoons (30 mL) drained capers

Juice of 1 lemon

1 can (14 ounces/398 mL) artichoke hearts, drained and chopped

2 cups (500 mL) asparagus cut diagonally in bite-size pieces

2 ounces (55 g) whole-grain pasta, cooked

2 tablespoons (30 mL) chopped fresh parsley

1. Heat a large nonstick sauté pan over medium-high heat. Add olive oil.
2. Add shallot; sauté until fragrant, about 1 minute.
3. Season chicken with salt and pepper. Add chicken to pan; cook, turning once, until cooked through and beginning to brown, about 3 minutes per side. Transfer chicken and shallots to a plate.
4. Return pan to heat. Add wine (if using), broth, capers, and lemon juice, scraping up any browned bits on bottom of pan.
5. Stir in artichokes and asparagus. Return chicken, shallots, and any accumulated juices to the pan. Cover and cook for about 5 minutes, until asparagus is tender-crisp.
6. Toss with cooked pasta. Divide between 2 dishes and sprinkle with parsley.

**Nutritional Information (per serving)**

Calories 378 • Carbs 45 grams • Protein 29 grams • Fat 9 grams • Fiber 12 grams

# Italian Sausage with Kale and Cannellini Beans

You won't believe you made this meal in 15 minutes—and neither will anyone else!  **SERVES 4**

Cooking oil spray

1 cup (250 mL) chopped onion

4 cups (1 L) halved cherry tomatoes

8 cups (2 L) chopped kale

Salt and pepper

1 cup (250 mL) fat-free chicken or vegetable broth

2½ cups (625 mL) canned cannellini beans, drained and rinsed

1 large pork Italian sausage or 2 chicken Italian sausages,
   casings removed, shredded or finely chopped

1. Heat a Dutch oven or soup pot over medium-high heat. Spray with cooking oil.
2. Add onions and tomatoes; sauté until tomatoes begin to caramelize and burst, about 6 minutes.
3. Stir in kale; cook until wilted. Season with salt and pepper.
4. Add broth, scraping up any browned bits. Stir in beans and sausage. Simmer until sausage is cooked, about 5 minutes. Adjust seasoning if needed.

**Nutritional Information (per serving)**

Calories 369  •  Carbs 58 grams  •  Protein 23 grams  •  Fat 7 grams  •  Fiber 15 grams

# SNACKS AND DIPS

# Lemon Parmesan Popcorn

Most store-bought or movie theater popcorns are loaded with butter, salt, and artificial ingredients. This popcorn is way more flavorful and nutritious.  **SERVES 2**

3½ cups (875 mL) air-popped popcorn
  (generous 2 tablespoons/35 mL kernels)

1 teaspoon (5 mL) extra-virgin olive oil

1 tablespoon (15 mL) freshly grated Parmesan cheese

1 tablespoon (15 mL) ground flaxseed

½ teaspoon (2 mL) lemon pepper

¼ teaspoon (1 mL) salt

1. Toss popcorn with oil.
2. Sprinkle Parmesan, flaxseed, lemon pepper, and salt over popcorn; toss to coat.

### Nutritional Information (per serving)

Calories 102  •  Carbs 12 grams  •  Protein 4 grams  •  Fat 5 grams  •  Fiber 3 grams

# Sweet Potato Mini Muffins

The sweet potato in these muffins adds a ton of sweetness but also major moisture. Look for sweet potato purée in the baby food section at the supermarket, or make your own: Bake 2 large or 3 medium sweet potatoes in a 400°F (200°C) oven for 1 hour. When cool, remove peel and purée flesh in a food processor or with a fork. **MAKES 45 MINI MUFFINS (3 per serving)**

Cooking oil spray

1½ cups (375 mL) old-fashioned rolled oats

1¼ cups (300 mL) whole wheat flour

1 teaspoon (5 mL) cinnamon

1 teaspoon (5 mL) baking powder

½ teaspoon (2 mL) baking soda

½ teaspoon (2 mL) salt

½ teaspoon (2 mL) stevia

2 large eggs

1½ cups (375 mL) unsweetened cooked sweet potato purée

¾ cup (175 mL) skim milk

¼ cup (60 mL) coconut oil or canola/vegetable oil blend

1 teaspoon (5 mL) vanilla extract

1. Preheat oven to 350°F (180°C). Spray a mini muffin pan with cooking oil or line with paper liners.
2. In a medium bowl, combine oats, flour, cinnamon, baking powder, baking soda, salt, and stevia.
3. In a large bowl, whisk eggs. Add sweet potato purée, milk, oil, and vanilla; whisk until well blended.
4. Gradually stir dry ingredients into wet ones just until blended—be sure not to overmix.
5. Divide batter among muffin cups. Bake for 12 to 15 minutes. To test for doneness, stick a toothpick into the center of a muffin. If it comes out dry, they're done. Turn muffins out onto a rack to cool. You may freeze the muffins for up to 3 months.

**Nutritional Information (per serving)**

Calories 140 • Carbs 20 grams • Protein 5 grams • Fat 5 grams • Fiber 3 grams

# Bacon Cheddar Veggie Muffins

This is an easy, classic snack to whip up.  **MAKES 15 MUFFINS (1 per serving)**

Cooking oil spray

4 slices reduced-fat bacon

5 cups (1.25 L) fresh spinach (12 ounces/ 340 g), chopped

1 cup (250 mL) diced zucchini

1 cup (250 mL) canned black beans, drained and rinsed

Salt and pepper

1 cup (250 mL) whole wheat flour

¾ cup (175 mL) all-purpose flour

¼ cup (60 mL) ground flaxseed

1 teaspoon (5 mL) baking powder

1 teaspoon (5 mL) baking soda

½ teaspoon (2 mL) salt

½ teaspoon (2 mL) ground cumin

2 large eggs

1½ cups (375 mL) skim milk

1 tablespoon (15 mL) olive oil

1 cup (250 mL) shredded low-fat Cheddar cheese

Chopped jalapeño peppers to taste (optional)

1. Preheat oven to 375°F (190°C). Spray a muffin pan with cooking oil or line with paper liners.
2. Heat a large sauté pan over medium heat. Cook bacon until crisp. Drain on paper towels. Crumble when cool.
3. While bacon cools, drain excess oil from pan, leaving a minimal amount in the pan. Add spinach, zucchini, and beans; cook just until spinach is wilted, 2 to 3 minutes. Stir in crumbled bacon. Season with salt and pepper.
4. In a large bowl, combine whole wheat flour, all-purpose flour, flaxseed, baking powder, baking soda, salt, and cumin; stir to blend.
5. In a medium bowl, combine eggs, milk, and olive oil; whisk until well blended.
6. Add egg mixture to dry ingredients; stir just until combined. Do not overmix.
7. Gently fold in cheese, spinach mixture, and jalapeños (if using) just until combined. Let rest for 5 minutes.
8. Fill each muffin cup three-quarters full. Bake for 15 to 18 minutes. To test for doneness, stick a toothpick into the center of a muffin. If it comes out dry, they're done. Turn muffins out onto a rack to cool.

**Nutritional Information (per serving)**

Calories 147  •  Carbs 19 grams  •  Protein 10 grams  •  Fat 6 grams  •  Fiber 3 grams

# Spinach-Stuffed Mushrooms

I love putting these out at gatherings with friends. They taste much too decadent to be healthy, but they are! **MAKES 24 MUSHROOMS** (8 per serving)

Cooking oil spray

¼ cup (60 mL) dry bread crumbs

½ package (10 ounces/284 g) frozen chopped spinach, thawed, excess water squeezed out

¼ cup (60 mL) soft goat cheese

2 large pieces roasted red pepper (about ½ cup/125 mL)

5 sprigs fresh parsley

1 teaspoon (5 mL) lemon zest

Salt and pepper

24 white button or cremini mushrooms, cleaned and stems removed

2 teaspoons (10 mL) grated reduced-fat Parmesan cheese

1. Preheat oven to 375°F (190°C). Spray a baking sheet with cooking oil.
2. In a food processor, combine bread crumbs, spinach, goat cheese, red pepper, parsley sprigs, lemon zest, and salt and pepper to taste. Pulse just until mixed.
3. Stuff each mushroom cap with spinach mixture. Place on baking sheet. Bake for 15 minutes or until top is lightly browned.
4. Sprinkle with Parmesan cheese and serve immediately.

**Nutritional Information (per serving)**

Calories 150 • Carbs 17 grams • Protein 11 grams • Fat 6 grams • Fiber 3 grams

# Butternut
# Black Bean Crostini

Making this snack makes me feel like a gourmet chef. It's delicious and beautiful, like a catered hors d'oeuvre. **MAKES 2 SERVINGS (4 per serving)**

8 slices (¼ inch/5 mm thick) whole-grain baguette

Cooking oil spray

½ cup (125 mL) chopped peeled butternut squash

Pinch of hot smoked paprika

Salt and pepper

½ cup (125 mL) fat-free or low-fat refried black beans

2 tablespoons (30 mL) crumbled feta cheese

Balsamic glaze or chopped fresh chives, for garnish

1. Spray baguette slices with cooking oil; toast in toaster oven (or broil) until just beginning to brown. Let cool.
2. Heat a small nonstick sauté pan over medium-high heat. Spray with cooking oil.
3. Add butternut squash; sauté until squash begins to soften and brown, about 5 minutes. Season with paprika and salt and pepper. Transfer squash to a plate.
4. Return pan to heat. Add black beans and stir until warm.
5. Spread black beans on each toasted baguette slice. Top with squash, followed by feta. Garnish with a few drops of balsamic glaze or a sprinkle of chives.

| Nutritional Information (per serving) |
| --- |

Calories 196 • Carbs 32 grams • Protein 9 grams • Fat 3 grams • Fiber 7 grams

# Pea and Parmesan Crostini

Fresh mint adds a touch of sophistication to this creamy and crunchy snack.  **MAKES 2 SERVINGS (4 per serving)**

8 slices (¼ inch/5 mm thick) whole-grain baguette

Cooking oil spray

½ cup (125 mL) fresh or thawed frozen peas

2 tablespoons (30 mL) finely chopped avocado

2 mint leaves, chopped

½ teaspoon (2 mL) lemon zest

½ teaspoon (2 mL) olive oil

Salt and pepper

1 tablespoon (15 mL) grated Parmesan cheese

Small fresh mint leaves, for garnish

1. Spray baguette slices with cooking oil; toast in toaster oven (or broil) until just beginning to brown. Let cool.
2. In a food processor, combine peas, avocado, mint, lemon zest, and oil; process until smooth. Season with salt and pepper.
3. Spread mixture on each toasted baguette slice. Sprinkle with Parmesan. Garnish each with a mint leaf if you're feeling fancy.

**Nutritional Information (per serving)**

Calories 146  •  Carbs 21 grams  •  Protein 7 grams  •  Fat 5 grams  •  Fiber 4 grams

# Chicken Sausage Pizza

For all you pizza lovers out there (I know there's a lot of you!), this pizza will satisfy your craving and appetite without the guilt.   **MAKES 2 SERVINGS (1 pizza per serving)**

½ chicken Italian sausage

¼ cup (60 mL) tomato sauce

2 low-carb high-fiber tortillas

½ cup (125 mL) shredded fat-free mozzarella cheese

Cooking oil spray

Hot pepper flakes to taste (optional)


1. Place a baking sheet in the oven and preheat oven to 400°F (200°C).
2. Grate sausage on the large holes of a box grater.
3. Spread half of the tomato sauce over each tortilla, spreading it to the edges. Sprinkle each with half of the cheese. Sprinkle with grated sausage.
4. Remove baking sheet from oven and spray with cooking oil.
5. Place pizzas on baking sheet. Bake until cheese has melted and tortilla starts to brown, 8 to 10 minutes.
6. Sprinkle with hot pepper flakes if desired. Cut each pizza into wedges.

**Nutritional Information (per serving)**

Calories 140  •  Carbs 15 grams  •  Protein 17 grams  •  Fat 5 grams  •  Fiber 8 grams

# Tomato and Green Olive Pizza

You won't believe that this topping-loaded pizza is only 140 calories.   **MAKES 2 SERVINGS (1 pizza per serving)**

¼ cup (60 mL) tomato sauce

2 low-carb high-fiber tortillas

½ cup (125 mL) shredded fat-free mozzarella cheese

1 cup (250 mL) halved cherry tomatoes

¼ cup (60 mL) green olives, pitted and chopped

Cooking oil spray

Hot pepper flakes to taste (optional)

1. Place a baking sheet in the oven and preheat oven to 400°F (200°C).
2. Spread half of the tomato sauce on each tortilla, spreading it to the edges. Sprinkle each with half of the cheese. Top evenly with tomatoes and olives.
3. Remove baking sheet from oven and spray with cooking oil.
4. Place pizzas on baking sheet. Bake until cheese has melted and tomatoes start to brown, 10 to 15 minutes.
5. Sprinkle with hot pepper flakes if desired. Cut each pizza into wedges.

**Nutritional Information (per serving)**

Calories 140  •  **Carbs** 18 grams  •  **Protein** 15 grams  •  **Fat** 4 grams  •  **Fiber** 9 grams

# Chicken Black Bean Nachos

When I say you won't miss out on anything on the Body Reset Diet, I'm not messing around. These nachos will please even the Sunday football crowd. **SERVES 4**

1 cup (250 mL) canned black beans, drained and rinsed

¼ cup (60 mL) fat-free chicken broth

2 teaspoons (10 mL) taco seasoning mix

Salt and pepper

Cooking oil spray

4 ounces (115 g) ground chicken breast

1 tablespoon (15 mL) water

24 baked or low-fat tortilla chips

½ cup (125 mL) shredded fat-free or low-fat Cheddar cheese

Canned jalapeño slices, drained (optional)

Chopped fresh cilantro, for garnish

1. Preheat oven to 400°F (200°C).
2. In a small saucepan over medium heat, warm beans with broth.
3. Add 1 teaspoon (5 mL) of the taco seasoning; mash with a wooden spoon. Season with salt and pepper.
4. Heat a small nonstick sauté pan over medium-high heat. Spray with cooking oil.
5. Add ground chicken. Break up chicken with a wooden spatula and cook until beginning to brown.
6. Add water, remaining 1 teaspoon (5 mL) taco seasoning, and salt and pepper to taste; stir to combine. Cook for 2 minutes.
7. Spread tortilla chips on a baking sheet. Top each chip with about 1 teaspoon (5 mL) of beans, then 1 teaspoon (5 mL) chicken. Sprinkle each with a pinch of cheese and top with a jalapeño slice (if using).
8. Bake until cheese has melted and chips just start to brown, about 4 minutes. Sprinkle with cilantro, if desired.

**Nutritional Information (per serving)**

Calories 165 • Carbs 21 grams • Protein 15 grams • Fat 2 grams • Fiber 4 grams

# White Bean Jalapeño Nachos

If fresh jalapeños aren't available, canned will work fine here.  **SERVES 4**

1 can (14 ounces/398 mL) cannellini or other white beans, drained and rinsed

½ cup (125 mL) fat-free vegetable broth

1 teaspoon (5 mL) ground cumin

1 teaspoon (5 mL) dried thyme

Salt and pepper

24 baked or low-fat tortilla chips

½ cup (125 mL) shredded fat-free or low-fat Cheddar cheese

½ cup (125 mL) chopped jalapeño peppers, seeded if desired

Chopped fresh cilantro, for garnish

1. Preheat oven to 400°F (200°C).
2. Combine beans and broth in a small saucepan; add cumin, thyme, and a pinch each of salt and pepper. Cook, stirring occasionally, over medium heat until liquid reduces, about 10 minutes. Mash half of beans with a wooden spoon. Stir in whole beans.
3. Spread tortilla chips on a baking sheet. Top chips evenly with bean mixture. Sprinkle chips with cheese and top with some jalapeño.
4. Bake until cheese has melted and chips just start to brown, about 4 minutes. Sprinkle with chopped cilantro, if desired.

**Nutritional Information (per serving)**

Calories 250  •  Carbs 25 grams  •  Protein 11 grams  •  Fat 1 gram  •  Fiber 4 grams

# Quinoa Cakes

These savory cakes are perfect for when you're craving a more substantial snack.  **MAKES 6 SERVINGS (2 per serving)**

3 cups (750 mL) cooked quinoa or other whole grains and/or beans

2 cups (500 mL) shredded zucchini (about 2 medium)

½ cup (125 mL) dry bread crumbs or panko

¼ cup (60 mL) egg whites (2 egg whites), lightly whisked

2 tablespoons (30 mL) grated reduced-fat Parmesan cheese

Salt and pepper

1 tablespoon (15 mL) coconut oil or other vegetable oil

Lemon wedges (optional)

1. In a medium bowl, combine quinoa, zucchini, bread crumbs, egg whites, and Parmesan; mix well. Season with salt and pepper. Using your hands, firmly pack mixture into 12 small cakes.
2. Heat a large nonstick sauté pan over medium-high heat. Add coconut oil.
3. Fry cakes until browned and crispy and cooked through, about 5 minutes per side. Cook covered to speed up cooking time, if desired. Serve with lemon wedges.

**Nutritional Information (per serving)**

Calories 190 • Carbs 31 grams • Protein 8 grams • Fat 5 grams • Fiber 4 grams

# Zucchini and Goat Cheese Involtini

These little bites taste and look good enough to serve at a wedding or fancy party, but they take only a few minutes to prepare. **SERVES 2**

Cooking oil spray

2 small zucchini, sliced lengthwise ¼ inch (5 mm) thick (4 to 5 slices per zucchini)

Salt and pepper

¼ cup (60 mL) fat-free cream cheese

2 tablespoons (30 mL) crumbled soft goat cheese

½ teaspoon (2 mL) lemon zest

½ teaspoon (2 mL) fresh or dried thyme

Balsamic glaze (optional)

1. Heat a medium nonstick sauté pan over medium-high heat. Spray with cooking oil.
2. Working in batches, add zucchini slices. Sprinkle with a pinch of salt and pepper. Cook, turning once, until zucchini begins to brown and soften, 3 to 4 minutes per side. Transfer to a plate and let cool.
3. In a small bowl, combine cream cheese, goat cheese, lemon zest, and thyme; mix together well. Season with salt and pepper.
4. Spread about 1½ teaspoons (7 mL) of cheese mixture on one side of each cooled zucchini slice. Starting from the narrower end, roll up zucchini. Top each with a drop of balsamic glaze, if desired.

**Nutritional Information (per serving)**

Calories 112 • Carbs 11 grams • Protein 8 grams • Fat 4 grams • Fiber 3 grams

# Quinoa-Stuffed Peppers

A trendy grain popularized for its balance of nutrients, quinoa is a healthy alternative to pasta and rice. It's all about keeping your meals interesting! **SERVES 2**

Cooking oil spray

¼ cup (60 mL) chopped onion

10 cups (2.4 L) fresh spinach (1 pound/450 g), chopped

½ cup (125 mL) cooked quinoa

½ cup (125 mL) fresh corn kernels

¼ cup (60 mL) diced tomatillos or tomatoes

¼ cup (60 mL) fat-free cream cheese, at room temperature

2 tablespoons (30 mL) chopped fresh cilantro

1 tablespoon (15 mL) lime juice

Salt and pepper

2 green peppers (poblano, pasilla, or bell), tops removed, seeded

1. Preheat oven to 425°F (220°C). Spray a baking sheet with cooking oil.
2. Heat a medium nonstick sauté pan over medium-high heat. Spray with cooking oil.
3. Add onions and spinach; cook, stirring often, until spinach is wilted and onions are soft, about 5 minutes. Transfer to a medium bowl.
4. Add quinoa, corn, tomatillos, cream cheese, cilantro, and lime juice; stir to combine. Season with salt and pepper.
5. Divide quinoa mixture between peppers. Place on baking sheet.
6. Bake for 15 minutes or until peppers soften. Serve hot.

### Nutritional Information (per serving)

Calories 201 • Carbs 36 grams • Protein 13 grams • Fat 3 grams • Fiber 8 grams

# Cali Tuna Salad with Crispbread

The creaminess of the avocado will have you forgetting that this recipe uses fat-free mayonnaise.
**SERVES 4**

8 ounces (225 g) canned tuna in water, drained

1 cup (250 mL) diced unpeeled apple

½ cup (125 mL) fat-free mayonnaise (or ¼ cup/60 mL reduced-fat mayonnaise)

⅓ cup (75 mL) diced dill pickle

¼ cup (60 mL) sweet pickle relish

Salt and pepper

¼ medium avocado, peeled and diced

4 Scandinavian high-fiber crackers (such as Wasa, Ryvita, Finn Crisp)

1. In a medium bowl, combine tuna, apple, mayonnaise, dill pickle, and relish; season with salt and pepper.
2. Serve topped with diced avocado. Serve with crispbread.

**Nutritional Information (per serving)**

Calories 163 • Carbs 24 grams • Protein 12 grams • Fat 2 grams • Fiber 4 grams

# Chili Con Queso

Once you try this dip, you won't go back to the neon orange stuff.  **SERVES 2**

¼ teaspoon (1 mL) olive oil

¼ cup (60 mL) finely chopped onion

½ clove garlic, chopped

½ cup (125 mL) + 1 tablespoon (15 mL) skim milk

1½ teaspoons (7 mL) cornstarch

½ cup (125 mL) shredded low-fat Cheddar cheese

½ cup (125 mL) canned tomatoes with green chili

1 teaspoon (5 mL) lime juice

⅛ teaspoon (0.5 mL) chili powder

Salt and pepper

1 tablespoon (15 mL) chopped fresh cilantro

1 tablespoon (15 mL) chopped green onions

12 baked or low-fat tortilla chips

1. Heat oil in a medium saucepan over medium heat.
2. Add onions and garlic; cook, stirring often, for 4 to 5 minutes or until onions are soft and starting to brown.
3. Add ½ cup (125 mL) of the milk. Bring to a simmer.
4. In a small bowl, whisk together cornstarch and remaining 1 tablespoon (15 mL) milk. Add to pan and whisk until combined. Cook, stirring, until bubbling and thickened, 1 to 2 minutes.
5. Reduce heat to low. Add cheese; stir until melted.
6. Stir in tomatoes, lime juice, and chili powder. Season with salt and pepper.
7. Serve topped with cilantro and green onions. Serve with tortilla chips.

**Nutritional Information (per serving)**

Calories 202  •  Carbs 27 grams  •  Protein 12 grams  •  Fat 5 grams  •  Fiber 4 grams

# Lemon Artichoke Dip with Crudités

This snack packs quite a punch for under 200 calories. You'll be satisfied for hours.  **SERVES 3**

1 can (14 ounces/398 mL) artichoke hearts, drained

¾ cup (175 mL) nonfat plain Greek yogurt

½ cup (125 mL) fat-free cream cheese

⅓ cup (75 mL) grated reduced-fat Parmesan cheese

¼ cup (60 mL) chopped fresh parsley

¼ cup (60 mL) low-fat sour cream, softened

1 clove garlic

Juice of 1 lemon

Salt and pepper

Hot sauce (optional)

15 medium baby carrots

8 medium celery ribs, cut into sticks

1 small English cucumber, cut into sticks

1. In a food processor or blender, combine artichoke hearts, yogurt, cream cheese, Parmesan, parsley, sour cream, garlic, and lemon juice; pulse until fully combined. Pulse longer for a smoother, creamier dip. Season with salt, pepper, and hot sauce (if using).
2. Serve with carrots and veggie sticks.

| Nutritional Information (per serving) |
| --- |

**Calories 183  •  Carbs 19 grams  •  Protein 16 grams  •  Fat 5 grams  •  Fiber 4 grams**

# Warm Spinach Dip with Whole Wheat Pita

Restaurant spinach dips are almost categorically terrible for you, but my healthy version leaves nothing to be desired! **SERVES 2**

Cooking oil spray

½ cup (125 mL) chopped onion

1 clove garlic, chopped

4 cups (1 L) fresh spinach (8 ounces/225 g), chopped

Salt and pepper

½ cup (125 mL) nonfat plain Greek yogurt

¼ cup (60 mL) fat-free cream cheese

2 tablespoons (30 mL) grated reduced-fat Parmesan cheese

Pinch of paprika

2 small whole wheat pita breads, toasted and cut in wedges

1. Heat a small saucepan over medium heat. Spray with cooking oil.
2. Add onions, garlic, and spinach; sauté until onions are soft and spinach is wilted, about 7 minutes. Season with salt and pepper.
3. Turn off heat and add yogurt, cream cheese, and Parmesan. Stir until warmed through. Season to taste with salt and pepper.
4. Transfer to a serving dish and sprinkle with paprika. Serve with toasted pita wedges.

| Nutritional Information (per serving) |
| --- |

Calories 189 • Carbs 24 grams • Protein 17 grams • Fat 4 grams • Fiber 4 grams

# French Onion Dip
# with Baby Carrots

Most store-bought onion dips are high in fat and full of unrecognizable ingredients (hydrolyzed torula? glucono delta-lactone?). My lighter version is much healthier and will definitely make your taste buds happy. **SERVES 2**

Cooking oil spray

1 cup (250 mL) chopped onion

1 teaspoon (5 mL) fresh thyme
(or ½ teaspoon/2 mL dried)

Salt and pepper

¼ cup (60 mL) fat-free beef broth

1 tablespoon (15 mL) Worcestershire sauce

½ cup (125 mL) nonfat plain Greek yogurt

⅓ cup (75 mL) fat-free sour cream

¼ cup (60 mL) low-fat cream cheese

24 baby carrots

1. Heat a medium saucepan over medium-high heat. Spray with cooking oil.
2. Add onions, thyme, and a pinch each of salt and pepper; cook, stirring occasionally, until onions are beginning to brown, about 5 minutes.
3. Add broth and Worcestershire sauce, scraping up any browned bits. Simmer until liquid is almost evaporated, about 4 minutes.
4. Reduce heat to medium-low and cook until onions are deep golden brown, about 7 minutes more. Remove from heat, spread on a plate, and cool in refrigerator for 10 minutes.
5. In a medium bowl, combine yogurt, sour cream, and cream cheese; stir until smooth. Stir in onion mixture. Serve with carrots.

### Nutritional Information (per serving)

Calories 208 • Carbs 31 grams • Protein 12 grams • Fat 5 grams • Fiber 5 grams

# Slimmed-Down Guacamole and Chips

Although I love avocados, the calories in guacamole can add up pretty fast—and I've never been able to stop myself at just a couple of tablespoons. So I came up with my own slimmed-down version. **SERVES 3**

8 medium asparagus spears, steamed, cooled, and cut in 1-inch (2.5 cm) pieces

½ cup (125 mL) fresh or frozen peas, steamed and cooled

½ medium avocado, peeled and sliced

¼ cup (60 mL) canned white beans (cannellini, Great Northern, or navy),
    drained and rinsed

2 tablespoons (30 mL) chopped fresh cilantro

2 tablespoons (30 mL) chopped red onion

1 tablespoon (15 mL) canned chopped jalapeño pepper
    (or 1 teaspoon/5 mL juice from can)

1 clove garlic

Juice of ½ lime

1 cup (250 mL) chopped seeded tomato

Salt and pepper

18 baked or low-fat tortilla chips

1. Place asparagus and peas in a food processor; pulse until finely chopped.
2. Add avocado, beans, cilantro, onion, jalapeño, garlic, and lime juice; blend to the desired texture. You can leave it chunky or process longer for a smooth purée.
3. Fold in chopped tomato. Season with salt and pepper.
4. Transfer to a serving dish and serve with tortilla chips.

**Nutritional Information (per serving)**

**Calories 180** • **Carbs 28 grams** • **Protein 7 grams** • **Fat 6 grams** • **Fiber 7 grams**

# Four-Layer Dip
# with Fiber Crispbread

I love Scandinavian crispbread. It's so crunchy and loaded with fiber. And this dip is as pretty as it is delicious! **SERVES 3**

½ cup (125 mL) canned black beans, drained and rinsed

½ cup (125 mL) fat-free salsa

Salt and pepper

½ cup (125 mL) fat-free sour cream

2 teaspoons (10 mL) taco seasoning mix

¼ cup (60 mL) diced seeded tomato

¼ cup (60 mL) chopped onion

1 tablespoon (15 mL) chopped fresh cilantro

¼ medium avocado, peeled and chopped

1 tablespoon (15 mL) lime juice

1 tablespoon (15 mL) crumbled cotija or other Mexican cheese

3 Scandinavian high-fiber crackers (such as Wasa, Ryvita, Finn Crisp)

1. In a food processor, combine black beans and salsa; process until smooth. Season with salt and pepper.
2. In a small bowl, stir together sour cream and 1 teaspoon (5 mL) of the taco seasoning until blended.
3. In another small bowl, combine tomatoes, onions, remaining 1 teaspoon (5 mL) taco seasoning, and half the cilantro; stir to combine.
4. In a third small bowl, stir together avocado, lime juice, and remaining cilantro.
5. Spread bean mixture evenly over bottom of a serving dish, followed by sour cream mixture, then tomato mixture, then the avocado. Sprinkle with cheese. Serve with crispbread.

### Nutritional Information (per serving)

Calories 156 • Carbs 25 grams • Protein 7 grams • Fat 4 grams • Fiber 6 grams

# SWEETS AND TREATS

# Power Cookie

I realize that cannellini beans might be a surprising ingredient here, but try it before you dismiss it. You won't be disappointed! You can make your own oat flour by blending rolled oats to a fine flour.

**MAKES 12 SERVINGS (2 cookies per serving)**

¾ cup (175 mL) canned cannellini beans, drained and rinsed

⅓ cup (75 mL) egg substitute

¼ cup (60 mL) stevia and brown sugar blend or Splenda and brown sugar blend

4 teaspoons (20 mL) coconut oil

1 teaspoon (5 mL) vanilla extract

1⅓ cups (325 mL) oat flour

¼ cup (60 mL) unsweetened flaked coconut

3 tablespoons (45 mL) ground flaxseed

½ teaspoon (2 mL) baking soda

½ teaspoon (2 mL) baking powder

½ teaspoon (2 mL) salt

½ cup (125 mL) dates, pitted and chopped

¼ cup (60 mL) raisins

1. Preheat oven to 350°F (180°C). Line 2 baking sheets with parchment paper.
2. In a food processor, process beans to a smooth purée, adding a small amount of water if needed.
3. Add egg substitute, sugar blend, coconut oil, and vanilla; pulse to combine.
4. In a separate bowl, combine oat flour, coconut, flaxseed, baking soda, baking powder, and salt; mix well. Stir in dates and raisins.
5. Add liquid ingredients to dry mixture, stirring until completely mixed.
6. Roll dough into 24 balls and arrange evenly on the baking sheets. Flatten with the palm of your hand.
7. Bake until just slightly golden brown on top, 12 to 15 minutes. Transfer cookies to racks to cool.

**Nutritional Information (per serving)**

Calories 143 • Carbs 25 grams • Protein 4 grams • Fat 4 grams • Fiber 3 grams

# Fruit and Nut Popcorn Bars

If you're craving a crunchy yet chewy treat, these bars are for you. They travel well in a sandwich bag.
**MAKES 20 SERVINGS (1 bar per serving)**

Cooking oil spray

7 cups (1.75 L) fat-free air-popped popcorn (6 tablespoons/90 mL kernels)

2½ cups (625 mL) bran buds cereal

2 cups (500 mL) old-fashioned rolled oats

½ cup (125 mL) raisins

6 tablespoons (90 mL) unsweetened shredded coconut

¼ cup (60 mL) ground flaxseed

24 raw almonds, chopped

10 dried apricots, thinly sliced

½ cup (125 mL) brown rice syrup

½ cup (125 mL) honey

1 tablespoon (15 mL) vanilla extract

⅓ cup powdered peanut butter (or 2 teaspoons/ 10 mL reduced-fat peanut butter)

¼ teaspoon (1 mL) salt

1. Preheat oven to 350°F (180°C). Spray a 13- × 9-inch (3.5 L) baking pan with cooking oil.
2. In a large bowl, combine popcorn, bran cereal, oats, raisins, coconut, flaxseed, almonds, and apricots; stir well.
3. In a small saucepan, combine brown rice syrup, honey, vanilla, peanut butter, and salt. Cook, stirring, over medium-low heat for 5 minutes.
4. Pour over popcorn mixture and stir until all ingredients are coated.
5. Pour mixture into the baking pan. Cover with wax or parchment paper (or use slightly wet hands) and firmly press mixture into baking pan.
6. Refrigerate for at least 2 hours before cutting into bars.

---

**Nutritional Information (per serving)**

Calories 187  •  Carbs 36 grams  •  Protein 4 grams  •  Fat 5 grams  •  Fiber 8 grams

# Baked Apples
# with Yogurt Custard

My wife makes these for us every week. They're just so good—they taste like a real treat and they make the whole house smell amazing!  **SERVES 4**

4 medium baking apples (such as Granny Smith, Honeycrisp, or Pink Lady)

1 cup (250 mL) nonfat plain Greek yogurt

¼ cup (60 mL) egg substitute

2 tablespoons (30 mL) cornstarch

1½ teaspoons (7 mL) vanilla extract

½ teaspoon (2 mL) stevia or sweetener of your choice

1 teaspoon (5 mL) cinnamon

⅓ cup (75 mL) all-bran cereal

1. Preheat oven to 375°F (190°C).
2. Cut the top off each apple. If necessary, trim the bottom so apples stand up. Using a melon baller or small spoon, scoop out the middle of each apple, leaving the bottom intact and leaving ½ inch (1 cm) flesh around the sides. Stand apples in a baking dish just large enough to hold them.
3. In a medium bowl, combine yogurt, egg substitute, cornstarch, vanilla, stevia, and half the cinnamon; beat until smooth. Stir in cereal.
4. Divide mixture among the apples, pouring to the top of each. Sprinkle with remaining cinnamon.
5. Bake until top is slightly browned, apples are soft, and custard is set, 30 to 40 minutes. Let cool for 10 minutes before serving.

---

**Nutritional Information (per serving)**

Calories 157 • Carbs 32 grams • Protein 8 grams • Fat 0 grams • Fiber 7 grams

# Mini Peach Custard

This delicious treat is best made in the summer when peaches are in season, as canned or frozen peaches don't work in this recipe. **SERVES 2**

Cooking oil spray

1 medium peach, pitted and chopped

¼ cup (60 mL) egg substitute

¼ cup (60 mL) skim milk

2 tablespoons (30 mL) cornstarch

¼ teaspoon (1 mL) vanilla extract

½ cup (125 mL) fresh blueberries

¼ cup (60 mL) old-fashioned rolled oats

1 tablespoon (15 mL) butter spread

½ teaspoon (2 mL) stevia or sweetener of your choice

1. Preheat oven to 375°F (190°C). Spray two ½-cup (125 mL) ramekins or ovenproof bowls with cooking oil.
2. Divide chopped peaches between ramekins.
3. In a medium bowl, whisk together egg substitute, milk, cornstarch, and vanilla. Stir in blueberries. Pour mixture over peaches.
4. In a small bowl, combine oats, butter spread, and stevia; rub together with your fingers until evenly mixed. Spoon mixture over peaches.
5. Place ramekins on a baking sheet and bake for 30 minutes or until custard is set. Let cool for 5 minutes before serving.

## Nutritional Information (per serving)

Calories 198  •  Carbs 30 grams  •  Protein 6 grams  •  Fat 6 grams  •  Fiber 3 grams

# Chocolate Banana Pudding

I'm definitely a huge fan of chocolate! This pudding satisfies my sweet tooth in a creamy, chocolaty, decidedly yummy way.   SERVES 3

1 banana, chopped

12 ounces (340 g) low-fat firm silken tofu

3 tablespoons (45 mL) cocoa powder

1 teaspoon (5 mL) stevia or sweetener of your choice

1 cup (250 mL) fresh raspberries

1.  In food processor, combine banana, tofu, cocoa powder, and stevia; process until smooth, at least 4 minutes.
2.  Divide pudding between 3 small bowls. Cover with plastic and cool in refrigerator for at least 20 minutes.
3.  Serve topped with fresh raspberries.

**Nutritional Information (per serving)**

Calories 174  •  Carbs 35 grams  •  Protein 9 grams  •  Fat 2 grams  •  Fiber 6 grams

# Acknowledgments

I want to thank …

Chef Sam McConell and Sarah Schier for helping me create these amazing recipes.

Allison Garfield for editing/coordinating/and anything else I could possibly need help with to make this book possible.

Andy Barzvi for convincing everyone I should get a fifth book published.

Andrea Magyar for making my home, Canada, the best place in the world to publish a book.

Laura Moser for helping me structure the words.

Shaun Oakey for helping me with the edits.

My amazing wife, Jess, for making me smile every day, all day.

# Index

BBQ chicken wrap, 127
chicken quinoa stir-fry, 155
cold Thai peanut noodles, 161
ginger and garlic tofu stir-fry, 154
steak and vegetable stir-fry, 160
tofu and greens soup, 143
calories, about, 2–3
cannellini beans. *See also* white beans
and chicken chili, 150
and Italian sausage with kale, 168
kale and chicken soup, 145
power cookies, 192
cantaloupe
and cucumber smoothie, 44
immunity boost smoothie, 69
carrot
Asian chicken salad, 114
beef stew, 151
chicken and vegetable soup, 144
coconut ginger smoothie, 84
cold Thai peanut noodles, 161
crudités, 185
and French onion dip, 187
hummus wrap, 126
kale and chicken soup, 145
miso chicken salad wrap, 128
pineapple cake smoothie, 73
spinach and apple smoothie, 59
spring vegetable salad, 118
tofu chickpea curry, 156
vegetable barley soup, 138
cashew, chicken, and vegetable stir-fry, 158
cauliflower soup, 148
celery
apple, quinoa, and blue cheese salad, 119
chicken and vegetable soup, 144
crudités, 185
kale and chicken soup, 145

chai tea smoothie, 85
cheese
bacon Cheddar veggie muffins, 172
blue, and apple and quinoa salad, 119
Cheddar and bacon topping for soup, 148
chili con queso, 184
lemon artichoke dip, 185
sandwich, grilled, 122
turkey, Brie, and apple sandwich, 124
cherries: antioxidant smoothie, 77
chia seeds, and pomegranate smoothie, 50
chicken
Asian salad, 114
barley burger, 133
BBQ chicken, 127
BBQ chili, 151
black bean nachos, 178
cashew and vegetable stir-fry, 158
cold Thai peanut noodles, 161
and egg hash, 100
grain salad, 116
grilled, and nectarine salad, 113
grilled, with bean salad, 117
Italian chopped salad, 120
and kale soup, 145
lemon caper, with artichokes and
    fettuccine, 167
pan roasted, with fennel and tomatoes,
    166
quinoa stir-fry, 155
salad and miso wrap, 128
sausage pizza, 176
sausage scramble, 91
in S-meals, 23
and spring vegetable salad, 118
sweet potato and kale soup, 146
taco salad, 115
and vegetable soup, 144

white bean chili, 150
chickpeas
    beef stew, 151
    coconut shrimp curry, 157
    Italian chopped salad, 120
    nectarine salad, with grilled chicken, 113
    open-faced vegetable scramble sandwich, 97
    as protein option, 24
    Spanish breakfast stew, 103
    Spanish chicken sausage scramble, 91
    spicy lentil burger, 131
    tofu curry, 156
    vegetable barley soup, 138
chilaquiles, 90
chili
    con queso, 184
    white bean chicken, 150
chocolate banana pudding, 196
cocoa
    banana peanut butter smoothie, 81
    candied almond smoothie, 86
coconut
    and apple smoothie, 38
    apricot banana smoothie, 41
    ginger carrot smoothie, 84
    mango smoothie, 68
    shrimp curry, 157
    spinach smoothie, 62
cod, miso, with spinach and sweet potatoes, 165
condiments in S-meals, 27
cookies: power, 192
corn kernels
    baked tofu summer salad, 107
    BBQ farro salad, 106
    chowder with edamame, 141
    quinoa-stuffed peppers, 182

salmon chowder, 142
shrimp salad, 108
smoked turkey spinach salad, 112
southwestern turkey burger, 136
white bean chicken chili, 150
cranberries
    grain salad, 116
    smoothie, 49
creamy green smoothie, 57
crostini
    butternut black bean, 174
    pea and Parmesan crostini, 175
C-snacks
    about, 7
    examples of, 28
cucumber
    apple smoothie, 66
    and cantaloupe smoothie, 44
    crudités, 185
    grilled salmon panzanella salad, 111
    Italian chopped salad, 120
    minty melon smoothie, 58
    miso chicken salad wrap, 128
    shrimp salad, 108
    watermelon orange smoothie, 64
custard
    peach, 195
    yogurt, 194

dairy goods. *See also* milk
    pantry suggestions, 32
dates
    power cookie, 192
    smoothie, 83
dressings
    for Asian chicken salad, 114
    for baked tofu summer salad, 107
    for chicken taco salad, 115

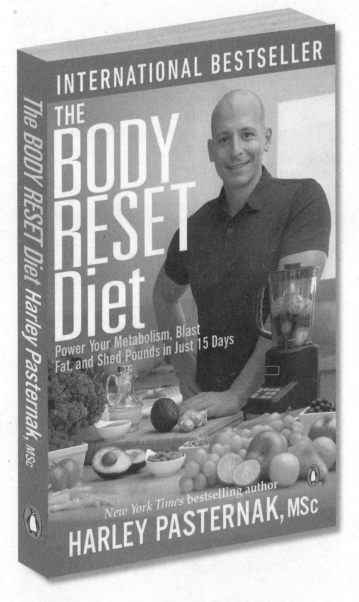

Whether you're looking to lose significant weight or just those last 5 pounds, *The Body Reset Diet* offers a proven program to hit the reset button, slim down, and get healthy in just 15 days—

## AND STAY THAT WAY FOR GOOD!

**AVAILABLE WHEREVER BOOKS ARE SOLD**

harleypasternak.com | @harleypasternak